HEALTH QUACKERY

Health Quackery

★ ★ ★ ★ ★ ★ ★ ★ ★

CONSUMERS UNION'S REPORT ON FALSE HEALTH CLAIMS, WORTHLESS REMEDIES, AND UNPROVED THERAPIES

The Editors of Consumer Reports Books

HOLT, RINEHART AND WINSTON / NEW YORK

Copyright © 1980 by Consumers Union of United States, Inc.,
Mount Vernon, New York 10550.
All rights reserved, including the right to reproduce this
book or portions thereof in any form.
This edition of *Health Quackery* has been published by
Holt, Rinehart and Winston, 383 Madison Avenue,
New York, New York 10017, by permission of
Consumers Union of United States, Inc.
Published simultaneously in Canada by Holt, Rinehart and
Winston of Canada, Limited.

Library of Congress Cataloging in Publication Data
Main entry under title:
Health Quackery.
1. Quacks and quackery. 2. Quacks and
quackery—United States. 3. Consumer protection—
United States. I. Consumers Union of United
States. II. Consumer Reports.
R730.H39 1981 615.8'56'0973 80-25777
ISBN Hardbound: 0-03-058899-5
ISBN Paperback: 0-03-058898-7

Health Quackery is a Consumer Reports Book published by Consumers Union, the nonprofit organization that publishes CONSUMER REPORTS, the monthly magazine of test reports, product Ratings, and buying guidance. Established in 1936, Consumers Union is chartered under the Not-For-Profit Corporation Law of the State of New York.

The purposes of Consumers Union, as stated in its charter, are to provide consumers with information and counsel on consumer goods and services, to give information and assistance on all matters relating to the expenditure of the family income, and to initiate and to cooperate with individual and group efforts seeking to create and maintain decent living standards.

Consumers Union derives its income solely from the sale of CONSUMER REPORTS and other publications. Consumers Union accepts no advertising or product samples and is not beholden in any way to any commercial interest. Its Ratings and reports are solely for the information and use of the readers of its publications.

Neither the Ratings nor the reports nor any other Consumers Union publications, including this book, may be used in advertising or for any commercial purpose of any nature. Consumers Union will take all steps open to it to prevent or to prosecute any such uses of its material or of its name or the name of CONSUMER REPORTS.

Printed in the United States of America
1 3 5 7 9 10 8 6 4 2

7059476

Contents

HEALTH QUACKERY

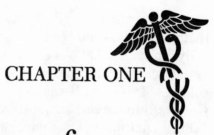

CHAPTER ONE

The Business of Health Fraud: Promising the Impossible

Quackery has existed, said Voltaire, since the first knave met the first fool. Perhaps the eighteenth-century French philosopher had the unicorn in mind. For centuries the legendary one-horned beast, which lived only in human imagination, was thought to be the source of a potent elixir. The horn of the unicorn was touted for epilepsy, impotence, barrenness, worms, the plague, smallpox, mad dog bites, and a variety of other complaints.

"In spite of the lack of the actual animal, the horn was usually available—at a price," wrote W. C. Ellerbroek in 1968 in *The Journal of the American Medical Association*. "Counterfeiting a valuable fake has always been worthwhile, and the ambitious were busy straightening walrus tusks and searching for other substitutes, such as the bones of domestic animals, stalactites, pieces of whalebone, and even limestone." According to Ellerbroek, "the value of the horns varied with the supply." At the peak of the market, pieces of unicorn horn and powder were said to have "brought up to ten times their weight in gold."

By Voltaire's day numerous patent medicines were being purveyed throughout Europe and the American colonies. Typically, Benjamin Franklin's *Pennsylvania Gazette* ran advertisements for the Widow Read's "Ointment for the Itch," which promised to drive away lice as well as "the most inveterate Itch." (The Widow Read was none other than Franklin's mother-in-law.) Quackery continued to prosper in America. In 1856 a pharmacist reported that scores of remedies were marketed "whose chief mission appear[ed] to be to open men's purses by opening their bowels."

Throughout the development of modern medicine, said this country's leading historian of quackery, James Harvey Young, Ph.D.,* "quackery's demise has often been predicted. This has certainly been so in America." Writing in *American Scientist* in 1972, Young went on to comment that Americans believed themselves to be "a reasonable people, and if error persisted here and there it would soon vanish because of our corporate good sense." Quackery "was acknowledged to be an evil but was considered transitory. When the populace had received a little more public schooling, when science had expanded its horizons a little further, or when Congress had enacted such-and-such a protective law, then would quackery vanish, consigned to the museum of outmoded delusions."

As democracy flourished, public schooling became a

---

*A professor of history at Emory University, Young is the author of *The Toadstool Millionaires* and its sequel, *The Medical Messiahs*.

virtual American birthright. Advances in medicine greatly expanded the ability of physicians to control or cure disease. And in 1906 Congress got around to passing the Pure Food and Drugs Act, which "required a modicum of accurate data on patent medicine labels," as Young put it. "As a result of the new act, *The New York Times* editorialized, 'the purity and honesty of the . . . medicines of the people are guaranteed.' The new law, exulted the *Nation,* would deal harmful nostrums a 'deathblow.' "

But, to paraphrase Mark Twain, the reports of quackery's death were greatly exaggerated. In fact, quackery thrived, despite wider opportunities for public education, the introduction of a host of medical and surgical advances, and the enactment of tougher laws during the New Deal years, which gave the federal government even more authority to crack down on flagrant forms of quackery.

According to the U.S. Food and Drug Administration, the term quackery encompasses both people and products: "The 'health practitioner' who has a 'miracle cure' but no medical training is a quack; the drug or food supplement promoted with false health claims is a quack product; the machine that has impressive knobs and dials, but does nothing except take money out of the pockets of the unsuspecting, is a quack device. Broadly speaking, quackery is misinformation about health."

Today, quackery is a multibillion dollar business, but the money wasted each year on quack products and treatments is only part of the problem. No one knows how many people have died of cancer because they

11

relied on quack treatments until it was too late for conventional therapy to be of help. Or how many arthritis victims have dissipated their life savings chasing false hopes—while their disease and disability grew worse. Or how many people respond to the blandishments of mail-order health quacks, thus abandoning reliable therapy for the dangers of unscientific treatment.

Some of quackery's hardy nostrums—bust developers, baldness remedies, weight-loss aids that "melt away" fat without dieting—are hawked largely through mail-order advertisements. But many quack schemes and products are promoted more subtly: in books, in magazine and newspaper articles, on radio and television talk shows, in the halls of Congress by skillful lobbyists—and even by members of Congress themselves. Food-fad remedies touted by self-appointed nutrition experts may euchre otherwise knowledgeable people as deftly as an ad for a bust developer or a hair restorer can fool the naive. Nor is quackery necessarily limited to practitioners without medical training. There are physicians who will provide unproved or irrational therapies—for a price. Other doctors may offer an unjustified medical diagnosis, with an expensive "treatment" to match.

Despite Voltaire's dictum, quackery has seldom been limited to transactions between knaves and fools. Indeed, the victims of quackery tend to come from all walks of life and educational backgrounds. Young noted that "few escape blindspots and areas of error that make them vulnerable to quackery under suitable circumstances. This goes for some . . . of mighty intellect with various degrees after their names."

It's not always easy to recognize a quack. Writing in the *Archives of Internal Medicine* in 1978, Stephen Barrett, M.D., a crusader against health deception, observed: "Most people think the modern health quack is easy to spot. But he isn't. He wears the cloak of science. He talks in 'scientific' terms. He writes with scientific references. And he is introduced on talk shows as the 'scientist ahead of his time.' The very word 'quack' helps his camouflage by making us think of an outlandish character selling snake oil. . . ."

If quack practitioners do not promote an FDA-regulated product or device along with their treatment, they can often operate beyond the arm of FDA authority. The FDA *can* take action if food, drugs, cosmetics, or medical devices sold in interstate commerce are misbranded or include false or misleading claims in their labeling. The agency can also act against such products if they are dangerous or, in the case of drugs, ineffective, and against products that are sold before complying with certain premarket requirements. Under current statutes, however, products that may be violating the law can be seized only after the FDA goes to court and only if the products are actually sold in interstate commerce.

The interstate commerce requirement also applies to the Federal Trade Commission, which is empowered to act against false and misleading advertising of over-the-counter preparations, but only if the product (or advertising) has first moved across state lines. The FTC has authority as well to seek an injunction to halt unfair or deceptive trade practices that are interstate in nature.

A third federal agency, the U.S. Postal Service, can

13

take action against anyone—including purveyors of quack products—who uses the mail to defraud. Proving a violation in court, however, has often been difficult, but recent changes in the law have increased the Postal Service's authority to deal with mail-order quackery. Now it has the power to seize or impound merchandise before final disposition of a case, including the period when appeals might be pending.

One might suppose that the three agencies together could do a reasonably good job of policing quackery. Each of them, however, has a relatively circumscribed area of authority and a heavy load of other responsibilities for a relatively small staff. In practice, it's usually very difficult to stop a determined peddler of questionable health products or services. The FDA spent more than a decade in the courts before the worthless Hoxsey cancer clinics closed down. In a classic case, it took sixteen years of litigation for the FTC to have the word *Liver* removed from *Carter's Little Liver Pills.* Moreover, state and local enforcement agencies are so poorly staffed that they can act only infrequently; and when they do, the offender may merely pay a fine—and move the operation elsewhere.

Because of the limited success of governmental efforts to halt deceptive health promotions, the need for consumer awareness of such practices is underscored. With this book, Consumers Union seeks to lift some of the camouflage from the most prevalent and persistent forms of health quackery. In the chapters that follow, we explore the promotion of worthless remedies for cancer and arthritis; the false claims made for chiropractic treatments, weight-reducing schemes, and vitamin E; the scare campaigns against water fluoridation; the misrepresentation of hypoglycemia as a widespread disease and of nutrition as a universal cure for what ails you; and the use of mail-order health schemes to defraud consumers.

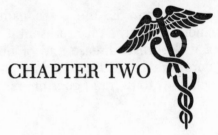

CHAPTER TWO

Laetrile: The Political Success of a Scientific Failure

Laetrile—an apricot-pit extract—was discovered quite by accident in 1920, its promoters claim, during an attempt to improve the flavor of bootleg whiskey. Supposedly "purified" in 1952, Laetrile has been struggling for respectability as a cancer remedy ever since.

Scientifically, it hasn't made it. But its political respectability has grown with stunning speed. State after state has passed laws legalizing its use. And a federal court ruled in 1977 that "terminal" cancer patients may receive Laetrile injections. That judgment was not upheld on appeal to the Supreme Court; neither was it struck down. In its June 1979 decision the nation's highest court did administer a wrist slap of sorts at Laetrile while remanding the case back to a lower court. But the proponents of Laetrile are far from conceding defeat. Instead they are increasingly turning to legislators who seem susceptible to the pressure group tactics used by the pro-Laetrile lobby. With Laetrile in legal limbo, the federal government's sixteen-year ban on the importation and interstate shipment of Laetrile could become obsolete. More important, the government's ability to rid the marketplace of quack remedies of all kinds may be jeopardized.

The power of political pressure is being felt even in the scientific world. Generally, major cancer research centers consider it unethical to test a drug on human beings unless it first shows promise in animals. Laetrile has shown no such promise. Nevertheless, the National Cancer Institute and the Memorial Sloan-Kettering Cancer Center—two organizations that have conducted extensive animal tests of Laetrile and found it ineffective—say that controlled human tests of Laetrile may now be necessary.

"Laetrile is a highly emotional issue that will not soon go away," an NCI official explained. "By conducting very careful human tests, we hope to prove once and for all time that the stuff is useless, and doesn't do anything that it's touted for." The NCI, in fact, applied late in 1978 to the U.S. Food and Drug Administration for permission to use Laetrile in clinical trials with humans and is awaiting the necessary clearances from the FDA for testing to begin.

A bill now before Congress would make such trials of drug efficacy very much beside the point. Under federal law, drugs must be proved safe and effective before they're marketed. But the "Medical Freedom of Choice" bill, which had more than one hundred representatives and senators as cosponsors when first introduced in 1977, would remove the necessity to prove a drug effective, requiring only that it be proved safe. An aide to Representative Steven Symms of Idaho, who sponsored the bill in the House, said that Laetrile had not been a factor in drafting the legislation. But the bill is strongly supported by pro-Laetrile groups. Its passage would immeasurably help their cause—and immeasurably damage some important consumer-protection safeguards in health and medicine. Besides removing the major obstacle to Laetrile marketing, such a law would legitimize countless other ineffective remedies as well. Representative Symms hopes to have hearings scheduled at some future date on a new version of the bill, the Food and Drug Reform Act. (A pro-Laetrile bill has also been introduced in Congress by Representative Larry McDonald of Georgia.)

Laetrile, a trade name coined by its developers, is the spiritual descendant of a long line of unproved cancer remedies, including such old-time "cures" as turpentine and green frogs and such twentieth-century hoaxes as Harry Hoxsey's herbal remedy and Krebiozen. In 1976 the American Cancer Society published a list of seventy-one self-proclaimed treatments promoted to help cancer sufferers but deemed valueless by the ACS. If the "Medical Freedom of Choice" bill becomes law, these products, or products like them, could flood the market. Costly and ineffective quack therapies could lure cancer patients away from anticancer therapies that might prove more medically effective.

Unlike the now-quaint quack cancer cures of past decades, Laetrile shows no signs of fading away on its own or being superseded by a new fad. Rather, the apricot-pit extract has rallied powerful political forces as well as some groups disenchanted with contemporary American life. Laetrile's appeal apparently touches a chord from an old American theme—rebellion at what seems to be arrogant inroads on individual freedoms by "big government."

Laetrile's appeal also plays on a more recent source of discord: anger at the "vested interests" of the "medical cancer establishment," which opposes Laetrile out of hand. Laetrile's promoters preach—and their followers believe—that the FDA is linked with "big business" (the pharmaceutical firms that manufacture anticancer drugs) and "big medicine" (the American Medical Association, the American Cancer Society) in a conspiracy to exploit the American people, especially the 400,000 or so who succumb annually to cancer. FDA cancer specialist Robert S. K. Young, a physician with a Ph.D. in pharmacology, observes that many cancer victims "are willing to try any and all nonrational magical solutions to the unsolvable problem of incurable illness." And many Americans disillusioned with the impersonal quality of modern health care or frustrated by the failure of a "can-do" culture to cure cancer seem willing to listen.

Moreover, the Laetrile lobby has broadened its appeal by attracting to its banners a number of other nonscientific, antimedical movements, notably the "orthomolecular" megavitamin cult for treating schizophrenia, those who tout the metal-chelating panacea for heart disease and the proteolytic enzyme cure for cancer, "organic" health food faddists, and opponents of water fluoridation. So Laetrile is not just this year's nostrum, being peddled by glib hucksters to naive or desperate people. Rather, it is the cutting edge of a concerted onslaught against established medical science and against the protection consumers now take for granted whenever they get their physicians' prescriptions filled.

When Laetrile was first discovered, its future impact could hardly have been foreseen. Derived from apricot pits, which contain cyanide, Laetrile was considered too toxic for human use by its discoverer, a Californian, Ernst Krebs, Sr., M.D. But years later, after his son, Ernst Krebs, Jr., claimed to have "purified" Laetrile, both father and son advocated it as an effective treatment for cancer. While Krebs, Sr., who died in 1970 at the age of ninety-three, had an M.D. degree, his son, Ernst, Jr., a medical school dropout, styles himself "doctor" on the strength of an honorary D.Sc. conferred upon him by a small Christian bible college in Oklahoma, an institution not accredited to grant advanced degrees to anyone. The Krebses patented their promising product as "Laetrile"—an acronym derived from the chemical name, *Lae*vo-mandeloni*trile*, the cyanide-containing substance they extracted from the crushed kernels of apricot pits. Thus was Laetrile off, if not yet running.

The next step was to explain how Laetrile worked. With a little imagination, the younger Krebs came up with a "magic bullet" theory. Cancer cells, he claimed, contain an abundant amount of an enzyme that releases cyanide from Laetrile. The cyanide, in turn, kills off the tumor cells. Normal cells are low in that enzyme, the Krebs theory went, but rich in another enzyme that detoxifies the cyanide. So normal cells live while cancer cells die.

That's an interesting theory—even potentially lifesaving, if right. But it's wrong. The supposedly abundant "releasing" enzyme is scarcer in cancer cells than in normal ones, and the "protective" enzyme is found in equal amounts in both kinds of cells. Moreover, cyanide does not have bulletlike precision. Because cyanide diffuses rapidly across intercellular barriers, any destructive effects would spread to both cancerous and noncancerous cells. Once that initial theory was discredited, Laetrile proponents shifted ground, suggesting a more complex sequence of biochemical events. Again, the scientific community found that the proposed mechanism had no validity. But the most dramatic and effective change in promotional strategy was yet to come.

After nearly two decades of unsuccessful attempts to get Laetrile approved as a drug, its promoters embarked on another course. Laetrile, the drug, was suddenly transformed in 1970 into Laetrile, the vitamin. Cancer, according to the later theory, was a vitamin-deficiency disease. Laetrile, it went on, was "vitamin B-17," the "missing vitamin" needed to prevent and treat cancer. As a vitamin and not a drug, Laetrile would be exempt from the stringent drug laws enforced by the FDA, including the requirement that a drug be proved safe and effective before it can be marketed.

Just one catch: Laetrile is not a vitamin. No disease, including cancer, has been associated with its lack in any animal. It is not an essential nutrient. It does not serve a unique bodily function, or, indeed, any bodily function at all.

The category change did not trick the FDA into looking the other way. As Consumers Union reported in the July 1974 issue of CONSUMER REPORTS, the FDA took legal action against *Aprikern* and *Bee-Seventeen,* two "health-food" products containing amygdalin, the commonly used chemical name for Laetrile. In 1975 a federal court in California placed the manufacturer of those products under permanent injunction. The judge found that "vitamin B-17" was not a recognized vitamin in human nutrition and that both products were actually adulterated foods. The next year, a federal court in New Jersey enjoined the distributors of *Bitter Food Tablets* from shipping the amygdalin-containing product across state lines. The court found that the promotion or sale of amygdalin as a food or drug constituted a fraud on the public.

While the vitamin ploy did not win over Laetrile's opponents, it did place Laetrile in step with the "health food" and megavitamin forces—forces that had already influenced government policy. In 1976 an active lobbying effort by these groups succeeded in severely curtailing the FDA's regulatory power over vitamin products.

Laetrile advocates no longer push "B-17" as an isolated therapy for treating cancer. Instead, Laetrile's promoters now present it as "the crown jewel in the diadem of total holistic metabolic nutritional therapy." This, they assert, can only be administered by properly trained "holistic metabolic physicians." Such training takes the form of weekend "doctors' workshops" held around the country, at which any medical doctor, doctor of osteopathy, chiropractor, druggist, or other "qualified" person can become such a "physician." Besides daily injections or oral doses of Laetrile, the "total holistic metabolic nutritional" regimen includes massive doses of vitamin C and other vitamins, chelated mineral supplements, even coffee enemas. In its latest form, the Laetrile-centered regimen emphasizes a strictly vegetarian diet, free of all animal protein. Often another nonvitamin, "B-15," or "pangamic acid," is prescribed. ("B-15" too is the creation of the same Ernst Krebs, Jr., who christened Laetrile "B-17.")

Today, cancer itself is no longer presented as Laetrile's sole target. "Laetrile does not pretend to treat or cure the lumps and bumps of cancer," states the movement's literature; rather, it helps the whole patient in unspecified ways to correct and to control the root cause of the tumor. In their literature, Laetrile promoters link cancer with what they describe as a spectrum of "degenerative killer diseases" allegedly caused by modern living's "pollution of air, water, food and mind." According to the new Laetrilite gospel, the first phase in this fatal process is "hypoglycemia," which is supposed to lead inexorably to emphysema, arthritis, atherosclerosis, heart disease, cancer, and death.

Laetrile is also promoted for the relief of cancer pain. Some patients report a feeling of well-being and decrease in pain with Laetrile use. But its action as a pain reliever has never been validated. Patients, however, often feel better if they and their doctors *believe* a particular treatment is beneficial, regardless of whether the treatment has any genuine effect. This phenomenon, which is known as "the placebo effect," has been shown to occur, on average, in about one-third of patients treated with dummy medication.

The history of Laetrile is thus a history of change:

changing theories, changing therapies, and most recently, changing claims. Instead of being touted as a cancer "cure"—a word no longer on the lips of most Laetrile promoters—Laetrile is now being hawked on other grounds. It purportedly "prevents" cancer, "relieves pain," "slows" or "controls" the cancer, promotes "euphoria." But what is the real story?

Laetrile is one of the most tested substances ever put forward as a remedy for cancer. In 1953 the Cancer Commission of the California Medical Association investigated Laetrile and found it ineffective. As part of that study, the commission discovered that all but one of forty-four patients treated with Laetrile still had an active form of cancer or were dead. A decade later, when the Cancer Advisory Council to the California State Department of Public Health reported that Laetrile had no value in treating or curing cancer, California banned the use of Laetrile. In 1965 investigators reporting in the *Canadian Medical Association Journal* found that two formulations of Laetrile—one manufactured in the United States and one in Canada—were both ineffective in cancer therapy.

The most comprehensive series of animal tests were done at Memorial Sloan-Kettering in New York City. From 1972 to 1976 approximately thirty-seven experiments were conducted using Laetrile on mouse and rat tumors. One researcher found evidence suggesting that Laetrile might inhibit the spread of tumors. But those results were not based on sufficiently sensitive techniques, and the findings could not be corroborated by other investigators. In all the other animal trials at the New York cancer center, Laetrile neither prolonged life, nor reduced tumor size, nor checked the spread of cancer. "Laetrile is not active against cancer," reported C. Chester Stock, Ph.D., head of the laboratory that conducted the experiments. "If something is active we would see it consistently active, which we have not seen with our Laetrile experiments."

Scientifically, Laetrile just doesn't get off the ground; but emotionally, it's flying high. An estimated 50,000 to 75,000 Americans take Laetrile. Reports circulate of miraculous cures with Laetrile. Although such testimonials are rich in dramatic impact, they lack scientific validity. Medical records submitted by Laetrile proponents have never substantiated the claims made. Many cancer patients who believe they've been cured by Laetrile find out later that they still have the disease. Others never had cancer to begin with. Some cancer patients have temporary remissions—periods when symptoms may actually improve; if Laetrile use coincides with such a remission, the patient may think Laetrile was the cause. In other instances, patients have taken Laetrile along with accepted medical treatment and then attributed their recovery partially or entirely to Laetrile.

In a search for objective evidence that Laetrile works, the FDA asked Ernesto Contreras, M.D., the head of a major Laetrile clinic in Tijuana, Mexico, to provide his most dramatic examples of success with the compound. He submitted twelve case histories, which the FDA evaluated in 1971–72. Only seven of the twelve case reports were fully documented, however. And all seven of the patients whose records were suitable for review had at some time received conventional cancer therapy in addition to Laetrile. As a result, any alleged improvements could not be clearly attributed to Laetrile.

A great deal of publicity about Laetrile has centered on "terminal" cases—patients with advanced cancer who turn to Laetrile as their last chance for life, or at least as a way to ease the pain. For them the issue seems to be hope, not scientific evidence—and the call for Laetrile legalization to uphold individual "freedom of choice" is compelling.

Such hope has been fostered by a folk hero of the Laetrile movement, Glen Rutherford of Conway Springs, Kansas, who won the first court decision allowing a cancer patient to import Laetrile for personal use. Rutherford was diagnosed as having rectal cancer in 1971. He refused surgery, choosing instead a trip to Tijuana for Laetrile therapy. Just fifteen days into his treatment there, his cancerous rectal polyp was cauterized—burned off—by Mexican surgeons. Surgical removal of a localized cancer early in the course of the disease may result in cure. Cancer specialists believe this to have been the case with Rutherford.

For several years after his return home, Rutherford continued to take Laetrile that had been smuggled into the United States and he attributed his survival and continuing robust health to Laetrile alone. When his supply of Laetrile dried up during an FDA crackdown on the smugglers, Rutherford brought the suit that won him celebrity and by its outcome gave large numbers of Americans legal access to Laetrile.

In December 1977 Federal District Judge Luther Bohanon in Oklahoma ruled that Glen Rutherford and other cancer victims certified "terminal" by a physician could import Laetrile despite the FDA's refusal to permit marketing of the drug. Under the judge's prior temporary order to the same effect, many doctors had been persuaded to sign such "Bohanon affidavits," and a brisk business sprang up around the legal importation of Laetrile from Mexico. Bohanon's decision, which overrode the safety and efficacy provisions of the U.S. Food, Drug, and Cosmetic Act was appealed by the FDA to the Tenth Circuit Court in Denver. That three-judge tribunal handed down its verdict in July 1978. "Safety" and "efficacy," it ruled, "have no reasonable application to terminally ill cancer patients," since for such people "there is no known cure"; hence, "Laetrile is as effective as anything else." The appeals court limited its authorization to "intravenous injections administered by a licensed medical practitioner to persons who are certified by a licensed medical practitioner to be terminally ill of cancer in some form." The decision seemed a clear victory for Laetrile.

In announcing his intention to challenge this decision in the Supreme Court, the then FDA Commissioner, Donald Kennedy, Ph.D., declared: ". . . it contains the remarkable finding that 'safety' and 'efficacy' do not apply to persons who are terminally ill. It would therefore deprive such persons of protection guaranteed to others under the terms of the Food, Drug, and Cosmetic Act."

In common with virtually the entire medical profession of the United States, Consumers Union's medical consultants found the Denver court's decision alarming because of the widening ripples of danger to which it exposed not only so-called terminal cancer patients but all consumers of medical care and medicines. The specific points of concern include the following.

□Putting physicians under pressure to certify cancer patients as "terminal"—thus making them eligible for Laetrile injections—would distort the time-honored obligation of physicians to continue a course of treatment for each patient to the best of their professional ability and ethical judgment, no matter how ill the patient seemed to be.

□Legalizing Laetrile injections would give the drug an aura of medical legitimacy—something that has eluded Laetrile on the basis of extensive animal tests. Laetrile supporters would be able to cite the fact that the drug was administered by such-and-such a physician in such-and-such hospital. As a result, Laetrile might take on the appearance of a viable alternative to proved cancer treatments, even though it had not earned that status in animal or human tests—procedures to which all other drugs are subject by law.

□Once Laetrile were allowed for "terminal" cancer, the pressure would mount to permit Laetrile at ever-earlier stages of treatment, on the seductive reasoning that if it's "good" for treating the last stages of the disease, it must be better yet given sooner—and no doubt best of all if taken as a cancer preventive. (Indeed, a leading Laetrile proponent has soberly suggested that people sprinkle some on their breakfast cereal every day.)

Increasing use of the Laetrile alternative might deter many cancer victims from accepting surgery, radiation, and chemotherapy. These conventional medical methods, against which Laetrile's promoters rail, do prolong life and do lessen suffering in an increasing number of cancers. Particularly in acute leukemia of childhood, choriocarcinoma, and Hodgkin's disease, and more recently in testicular cancer, radiation and chemotherapy can bring about virtually complete, long-lasting remission—cure, for all practical purposes—in a high proportion of the victims.

The issue of effectiveness is only one part of the Laetrile controversy. A change in emphasis by Laetrile supporters began in 1972 when John Richardson, a California physician with a large Laetrile practice, was arrested on charges of violating the state's cancer quackery laws. His first trial resulted in a conviction; that ruling was overturned on appeal, and two subsequent retrials ended in hung juries. But the defendant's legal situation had reverberations beyond the courtroom. Richardson belonged to the John Birch Society, and many of his fellow members had united in his support. One of them, Robert Bradford, turned the ad hoc defense group into an organization working for legalization of Laetrile—the Committee for Freedom of Choice in Cancer Therapy. That group, which claims 450 chapters and 23,000 members, leads the legalization fight. The major thrust of the group's argument is that the government should not interfere with an individual's choice of therapy, particularly if that therapy is without toxic side effects and is therefore "safe."

Laetrile's much-touted "harmlessness" was not at first strenuously contested by the government. Only after the 1977 court decision made the substance legally available to many Americans did the FDA begin to subject it to systematic toxicological study. The FDA's pharmacological analysis in 1977 indicated that Laetrile smuggled or imported from Mexico in the form of oral doses and vials of injectable material under the names "Laetrile" and "amygdalina" were potentially lethal sources of cyanide. What's more, vials of injectable amygdalin were found to be contaminated with bacteria and fungi. Ironically, laboratory tests hinted that amygdalin might even be cancer-causing in its own right.

Jerry P. Lewis, M.D., chief of oncology and hematology at the University of California School of Medicine in Davis, reported late in 1977 the case of a seventeen-year-old in Los Angeles who swallowed approximately 10½ grams (one-third of an ounce) of injectable Laetrile. The young woman had a convulsion ten minutes later and died without recovering consciousness. In mid-1977 a ten-month-old girl died in an upstate New York hospital a few days after gulping down several Laetrile tablets. Beyond these documented deaths, the FDA toxicologists suggest that many cancer patients whose death after long-term, high-dose Laetrile medication was attributed to their malignancy actually succumbed to slow cyanide poisoning from Laetrile.

An FDA Drug Bulletin, issued to all physicians, commented in 1977: "No worthless drug is without harm; a patient's choice of Laetrile to the extent that such choice delays or interferes with swift diagnosis and prompt effective treatment is potentially fatal."

Early diagnosis is important in most cancers, and swift treatment with such recognized therapies as radiation, surgery, and drugs offers the best hope for improvement and possible cure. Since cancer is often a progressive illness, any loss of time can imperil such efforts.

Unfortunately, each of the proved methods of cancer treatment may involve some discomfort or pain. Laetrile promoters constantly hammer at the theme that "Surgery slashes," "Radiation burns," and "Chemotherapy poisons." In comparison, Laetrile is touted as a pleasant, risk-free way of "treating" cancer.

If Laetrile is taken instead of proved remedies, it presents the ultimate risk. The FDA's Young has compiled a list of twenty-three cancer patients who switched from conventional medical treatment to Laetrile and subsequently died. The seventeen females and six males, ranging in age from four to sixty-five, "were as much victims of 'harmless' Laetrile as if the drug itself has poisoned them," Young asserted. His case histories include the following.

☐A four-year-old girl with embryonal rhabdomyosarcoma had been treated—and her cancer controlled—with combined chemotherapy from August 1975 to September 1976. Her parents then stopped the treatment and had her started on Laetrile plus enzymes and vitamins. "The patient was brought to the hospital," Young reported, "dead on arrival with aggressive widely infiltrating tumor."

☐William A. Nolen, M.D., chief of surgery at a county hospital in Minnesota, diagnosed early treatable cancer of the uterus in a thirty-five-year-old mother of three and recommended surgery or radiation. Instead, she went to Mexico and spent $3,000 on Laetrile treatment. When she returned to Nolen six months later, the cancer had spread to her pelvis, bladder, and rectum. She died one month later.

☐A fifty-eight-year-old woman came to surgeon Robert Lee Marsh of Glendale (California) Adventist Hospital with a lump in her left breast. She refused to have a biopsy. Five months later, when the lump had grown and surgery was imperative, she failed to keep an appointment to enter the hospital. Instead she saw the leading dispenser of Laetrile in northern California, John Richardson, whose medical license was later rescinded. "After spending $3,500 for Laetrile injections and tablets," Young related, "the woman returned to southern California and treated herself with apricot pits, which . . . produced two episodes of cyanide poisoning. In October 1976 the woman returned to Dr. Marsh. The tumor had taken over her entire left breast and was hemorrhaging so badly she required blood transfusions. At this point, the cancer was inoperable."

☐Richard Kaplan, M.D., a Florida oncologist, described the case of a twenty-year-old in Tampa whose cancer of the testicle had metastasized to his lung. This type of tumor, Kaplan pointed out, is particularly responsive to chemotherapy and is highly curable. Yet the youth's mother took him off chemotherapy in favor of Laetrile. When his metastases multiplied, the patient became frightened, resumed conventional treatment, and "responded again the second time around." Then his mother took him back to Laetrile and, reported Kaplan, "this young man died. . . ."

For all of Laetrile's scientific absurdity as an anticancer drug, a number of leading American medical specialists have come to believe that only controlled clinical (that is, human) trials under government sponsorship can once and for all demonstrate convincingly to the public the worth—or worthlessness —of the drug. The National Cancer Institute has been under some pressure to begin testing with human beings—a step that has never officially been done for Laetrile.

Before launching such a problematical clinical trial, the NCI decided to survey Laetrile's medical track record among some of the thousands of stricken Americans who have been treated with the drug clandestinely or legally in recent years. Early in 1978 the NCI sent a letter to 385,000 physicians and 70,000 "health proponents" in the United States, inviting them, with all due safeguards of patient confidentiality, to submit case histories of amygdalin's actual medical results. These reports would describe patients whose cancer had been unequivocally diagnosed, and who had taken no conventional therapy for at least thirty days before starting on Laetrile so that the latter's effects might be clearly evaluated.

The mass mailing yielded reports of just ninety-three cases; twenty-six of these were discarded because they contained too little information for evaluation. The panel of cancer specialists convened by the NCI to review the remaining sixty-seven case histories eliminated another eleven that presented incomplete data. The panel found that seven patients who had been reported as benefiting from Laetrile actually had experienced progression of their malignancies; nine others had their condition stabilize; two enjoyed complete remission and four partial remission. The panel set aside the remaining thirty-four because they had been treated with conventional forms of therapy along with their Laetrile, making it impossible to tell what it was that had helped them. Overall, the mailing provided no persuasive evidence of Laetrile's effectiveness.

Meanwhile, the NCI application for clinical testing is still pending with the FDA, as of this writing. Consumers Union's medical consultants believe that the NCI proposal represents capitulation to pressure and a setback for science. Laetrile should not be exempt from the established testing schedule for experimental new drugs: animal toxicity and dosage studies to measure safety and efficacy, followed by clinical trials with human patients only after a new drug has been shown to have a favorable risk-benefit ratio. None of the research centers that have conducted animal tests with Laetrile over the last five years or so has reported anti-tumor activity for the drug. Laetrile's dismal record in animal testing clearly does not warrant human trials. Moreover, to give Laetrile experimentally to human cancer patients and then compare its effects with conventional treatment given to other similar patients would raise an unprecedented moral and ethical dilemma. Not only would such a trial expose patients to a substance of dubious benefit and possible danger, but by the same token it would deny them accepted drugs of proved therapeutic value.

One leading cancer specialist who also opposes the NCI trials is James F. Holland, M.D., chief of neoplastic diseases at New York's Mount Sinai Medical Center. (Years ago Holland helped explode the myth that

Krebiozen cured cancer.) "No scientific protocol for a trial of amygdalin therapy in cancer patients would prove anything to the Laetrilists and their duped public," Holland contends. "They insist it can only be administered along with a wide spectrum of other unorthodox treatments—megavitamins, enzymes, coffee enemas, special diets, etcetera—supposedly tailored to the individual patients by practitioners indoctrinated in 'holistic metabolic medicine.' Before the test was finished, they would predictably cry 'Foul!' and would use the failure of the trial as evidence of a conspiracy to deny Laetrile its 'rightful place.' "

But what about the right to hope? Even if a drug has no proved value, might it not have psychological benefit for a terminally ill cancer patient? In the debate over Laetrile, legislators have repeatedly confronted the FDA with that question. In a typical exchange, one New York State legislator put it this way: "When you drive your car out of a car wash, doesn't it seem to run better?" Replied the FDA official: "Maybe, but my car would really run better if it had an engine job. And if anyone tells you a wash will improve your car's performance, he's committing fraud."

Consumers Union believes that the use of Laetrile as a treatment for terminally ill cancer patients stands in blatant violation of the basic patient right not to be duped and not to be offered a false sense of hope. Some people who realize that Laetrile is worthless nevertheless argue that the terminally ill are in a special category and should have the right to choose whatever therapy they prefer. But these patients also have the right to responsible, honest medical care of high quality for as long as they live. Dying patients rarely, if ever, require deceptive drug treatment.

Indeed, in its June 1979 ruling on Laetrile, the Supreme Court explicitly rejected the idea that laws requiring drugs to be safe and effective have no meaning for "terminal" cancer patients. It declared that "effectiveness does not necessarily denote capacity to cure. In the treatment of any illness, terminal or otherwise, a drug is effective if it fulfills . . . its sponsors' claims of prolonged life, improved physical condition, or reduced pain." According to the court, "For the terminally ill, as for anyone else, a drug is unsafe if its potential for inflicting death or physical injury is not offset by the possibility of therapeutic benefit." The opinion also noted that "with diseases such as cancer, it is often impossible to identify a patient as terminally ill except in retrospect."

In addition to being deceived, the patients or their families have to pay dearly for the deception. Laetrile therapy does not come cheap. The cost of a month's treatment at a Mexican clinic has been estimated at between $1,500 and $2,500. Laetrile smuggled into the United States is priced as high as $50 for a half-ounce vial for injection, compared with a $9 price tag in Tijuana. Tablets sell for nearly two dollars in this country, but cost only about three cents to manufacture.

That a lot of money made from Laetrile has been concentrated in just a few hands was brought to light in mid-1976 when eight Americans, one Canadian, seven Mexicans, and three Mexican firms were indicted on 171 counts of smuggling Laetrile into the United States. The indictment noted that Richardson, the California physician whose earlier prosecution and medical license revocation in 1976 had aroused the John Birch Society, banked more than $2.5 million for Laetrile treatments given over a twenty-seven-month period. Contreras, the Mexican physician with a Laetrile practice in Tijuana, deposited almost $2 million in bank accounts in San Ysidro, California, during that same time span. In addition, the indictment claimed, Robert Bradford, who organized the nationwide Freedom of Choice group, had received $1.2 million for seven hundred shipments of Laetrile. (Four of the Americans, including Bradford and Richardson, were convicted in April 1977 in the smuggling case. They got off with relatively light fines and suspended sentences. None of the other defendants ever came to trial.)

While some people undoubtedly support Laetrile for the money to be made, many proponents are true believers in the drug. Anger, bereavement, and frustration over the fact that cancer continues to claim so many lives, despite billions of research dollars earmarked for the "war on cancer" in this decade, help explain the apparently irrational support that Laetrile attracts.

Other supporters of Laetrile are committed to the political idea that less government is better government. The Committee for Freedom of Choice in Cancer Therapy, the largest pro-Laetrile organization, emphasizes constitutional rights and freedoms and denounces the medical establishment and government intervention in private affairs. Two other organizations fighting for Laetrile legalization are the International Association of Cancer Victims and Friends, and the

Cancer Control Society. The oldest of the pro-Laetrile groups is the National Health Federation, which has since 1955 championed unorthodox or unproved medical treatments. Several of its founders had been convicted of such offenses as misbranding dietary products, marketing electrical devices with false claims, or practicing medicine without a license.

Laetrile supporters have developed into a highly vocal and extremely effective political force. They sponsor conventions for cancer victims and their families. They distribute literature. They petition Congress and lobby for pro-Laetrile legislation. In Indiana hundreds of Laetrile backers were bused to legislative hearings to argue for their cause; their efforts paid off. The Indiana legislature overrode a governor's veto in 1977, making that state the first to legalize the manufacture and sale of Laetrile. Also overriding their governor's veto, Illinois's legislators endorsed the controversial cancer remedy in 1977.

But New York did not take the same path. When in 1978, for the second straight year, Governor Hugh Carey vetoed a pro-Laetrile bill passed by an overwhelming vote, he denounced the substance as "a step backward into medical quackery of yesteryear." The bills he refused to sign, he said, would have permitted Laetrile to be purveyed "with impunity by the unscrupulous for treatment of hearing loss, acne, obesity, mental condition or any other ailment." In 1979 Carey once again vetoed a pro-Laetrile bill. And California has rebuffed legalization of the apricot-pit extract two times.

A Massachusetts state representative, A. James Whitney, who had formerly supported legalization of Laetrile, denounced Laetrile promoters in 1978 as "charlatans and scoundrels." The 1978 pro-Laetrile bill died in committee after Whitney warned that if Massachusetts, "the Athens of medicine," endorsed it, other states might take similar action. He called treating cancer with Laetrile "mass murder." All told, as of mid-1979, twenty-one states have accorded legalization some degree of acceptance and bills in Laetrile's favor were pending in at least four other states.

By approaching the issue state by state, Laetrile proponents hope to bypass federal food and drug laws under which interstate shipment of a drug is prohibited unless its safety and efficacy has been proved to the FDA. The FDA does have the authority to nullify much of the intent of newly passed state legislation sanctioning use of Laetrile where there is an interstate aspect to the traffic in Laetrile. But that authority would be short-lived if a version of the "Medical Freedom of Choice" bill should become law. It would annul the FDA's present power to ban drugs whose medical efficacy cannot be proved, thus opening the door wide to marketing of Laetrile and other worthless nostrums across the country.

The emotional push to legalize Laetrile has moved some thoughtful people, including physicians, to believe that little or no harm may come from accepting the pleas of terminally ill patients or their families for a worthless drug. But the issue is not so simple. During the past seven decades, Congress has passed increasingly tough drug laws to protect consumers from the purveyors of quack remedies. Such laws could be jeopardized by the pro-Laetrile forces and by the state legislatures that bow to their demands. In CU's opinion, approval of Laetrile as an anticancer drug could devastate the carefully structured consumer-protection drug laws enacted in modern times and could open the door to the legitimization of quackery. According to the evidence on hand, Laetrile has no place in medicine's pharmacopeia.

Even more important, legislation like the "Medical Freedom of Choice" bill should have no place among the laws of the land. Such legislation would turn the clock back to a time when purveyors of worthless nostrums could freely prey on an unprotected public, exploiting the fears of the sick and the desperation of the dying. The fight against charlatans in medicine has been long and hard, and it is far from over. If the political victories of Laetrile turn the battle around, it is a more dangerous drug than anyone has imagined.

Editors' Note: In January 1980, the FDA gave permission to the NCI to begin tests of Laetrile on cancer patients. The FDA specified that preliminary tests for toxicity must be conducted prior to full-scale clinical trials. In February 1980, the federal appeals court in Denver held that Laetrile was not exempt from the need to prove safety and efficacy and that government requirements concerning Laetrile did not violate any rights of the terminally ill to choose their own medications. The ruling would appear to undermine the legality of "Bohanon affidavits" (see page 27).

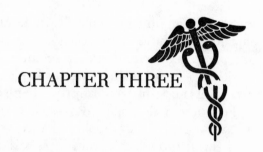

CHAPTER THREE

The Mistreatment of Arthritis

The only well-preserved spine of Neanderthal man is bent from arthritis. But when the first Neanderthal bones were discovered in 1856, treatment for arthritis had still not advanced beyond the cave era. In the 1850s Americans with arthritis could choose among some fifteen hundred advertised cure-alls, but the ingredients were usually flavored water, alcohol, narcotics, or toxic substances. Today, there is still no cure for arthritis.

Because quackery thrives best on human illness for which there is no cure, today's victims of arthritis and related diseases—nearly 32 million Americans—continue to be prime targets of hucksters, miracle-cure promoters, and charlatans. According to the Arthritis Foundation, a nonprofit national health organization, the current annual bill for unproved or quack arthritis remedies is an estimated $950 million.

Fortunately, many arthritis victims who once would have faced the prospect of chronic pain and eventual

41

disability can now be helped by a number of drugs and surgical techniques. But quackery has kept pace. For every dollar earmarked for scientific research in arthritic diseases, another twenty-five dollars is spent on worthless nostrums and unproved or irrational "cures."

For some patients, the outlay for various food supplements, wonder-diet books, folk remedies, liniments, and miracle devices is merely a waste of money. For others, however, the consequences are more serious. Some quack regimens are inherently unsafe. Others, while innocuous in themselves, may lead the arthritis victim to delay seeking proper treatment or to give up on medically prescribed therapy that takes effort and patience to follow. The result may be irreversible damage that could otherwise have been avoided.

Early diagnosis and sustained treatment can frequently prevent much of the pain and disability caused by rheumatoid arthritis, one of the most serious forms of the disease. Yet, according to the Arthritis Foundation, people with rheumatoid arthritis tend to wait an average of four years after symptoms first appear before seeking medical help. Often a factor in such delay is reliance on self-medication with over-the-counter products, home remedies, and the offerings of quacks. Ignorance about arthritis—and what should and should not be done for it—can be the arthritis sufferer's greatest handicap. Accordingly, in this chapter we will examine some of the basic facts about arthritis, including various forms the disease can take, some typical quack promotions, and the major methods of treatment that can genuinely help the majority of people with arthritic diseases.

The word arthritis literally means inflammation of a joint. But arthritis is actually many diseases—some mild, some severe. Approximately one hundred different ailments come under the heading of arthritis (or rheumatism, a term often used for vague unexplained aches and pains). All of them are characterized by pain in the joints and muscles. The more severe forms also show evidence of inflammation (redness, heat, and swelling) as well as pain, and they may affect other parts of the body besides the joints and muscles.

The cause of one form of arthritis can be entirely different from that of another. Quite different, too, may be the course of the disease and its treatment—facts that purveyors of catchall remedies commonly ignore. Some types of arthritis arise from still unexplained inflammatory processes. Others are caused by the degenerative effects of aging, by severe or repeated injury to a joint, or even by certain infections. Acute inflammation of one or several joints, for instance, may occur with bacterial infections caused by gonococci (the organisms responsible for gonorrhea) or staphylococci, but prompt antibiotic treatment can cure the infection and prevent severe joint damage. For most forms of arthritis, however, there is no cure. But the disease can be controlled, and its effects minimized, by proper treatment. The most important step in the control process is diagnosing the specific form of arthritis involved —as early as possible—so that treatment can begin before permanent damage occurs.

The most widespread kind of arthritis is osteoarthritis, or degenerative joint disease. Although sometimes capable of causing acute joint inflammation, it is primarily a "wear-and-tear" disease. It most frequently affects the large weight-bearing joints, such as the hips and knees, thus often causing pain on walking. Approximately 16 million people in the United States require some medical care for osteoarthritis. Although the ailment is usually mild, it can be severe in some cases. Nearly all people get at least a touch of osteoarthritis if they live long enough. Since the ailment generally occurs after the late fifties, some authorities believe it to be part of the aging process. (One exception is arthritis of the fingertip joints. Swellings called Heberden's nodes may appear over the end joints of the fingers in some people in their mid-forties.)

Another common joint disease is rheumatoid arthritis, an inflammatory form of arthritis that affects an estimated 6.5 million adults. It tends to be a recurring process, causing pain, swelling, and, in some cases, deformities in many joints of the body, especially in the knuckles and middle joint of the fingers. The disease usually starts between ages twenty and forty-five, affecting about three times as many women as men. A similar disease, juvenile rheumatoid arthritis, currently afflicts about 250,000 children. It can begin at any age from infancy through the teens. One form erupts suddenly, may affect internal organs, and can be severe. A second form comes on gradually, is milder, and is more likely to go away eventually. In both the adult and childhood forms, medical treatment can usually relieve symptoms and prevent or minimize disability. And the disabilities that do occur can often be modified by surgery. Nevertheless, people with rheumatoid arthritis can be easy targets for quacks. One reason is that the disorder is subject to periods of remission during which pain spontaneously subsides and symptoms disappear. If the improvement happens to coincide with the use of an unconventional remedy, the patient may think the treatment "cured" the disease. Such experiences are the basis of many sincere testimonials for worthless products or therapies.

The third most frequent arthritic ailment is gout, which affects an estimated 1.6 million people. An acutely painful inflammation, it most commonly strikes the large joint of the big toe, but it can also start in the knee, ankle, or some other joint. The majority of victims are men. In chronic gout, the accumulation of uric acid crystals in some joints may be disfiguring as well as disabling. Recurrent kidney stone attacks can also occur with chronic gout. The course of gout can vary from a few attacks in a lifetime to a progressive disease that begins at puberty and cripples its victims by the age of forty. Fortunately, effective treatment is available for both the acute and chronic forms of gout. Modern therapy can relieve or prevent pain and virtually eliminate the danger of crippling.

Among other forms of arthritis, four tend to be the most prevalent. One is ankylosing spondylitis, or arthritis of the spine, an inflammation that commonly strikes males in the teenage years or in the twenties, resulting in stiffness and sometimes deformities of the spine. Also called Marie-Strümpell's disease, it affects about one to two persons in every thousand. Another that occurs with comparable frequency is systemic lupus erythematosus, which can affect the skin and internal organs as well as the joints. It afflicts five times as many women as men. Commonly called lupus for short, the disease can usually be controlled, although in severe cases it can be life-threatening. (A mild form of lupus, which affects the skin only, is called discoid lupus erythematosus.) Arthritis of the fingertip joint may plague psoriasis sufferers. Patients with inflammatory bowel disease, such as ileitis, may also experience painful arthritis of the finger joints.

Localized ailments, bursitis and tendinitis, are common causes of musculoskeletal complaints. Both involve the joint area but unlike arthritis, which attacks the joint itself, bursitis and tendinitis affect structures surrounding the joint—the bursae and tendons. The inflammation usually arises from sprain, injury, or wear-and-tear damage. Bursitis attacks tend to be acutely painful but relatively brief, lasting only a week or two. Tendinitis is often less painful than bursitis but more persistent. With both, the overwhelming number of cases involves the shoulder. But other joints are also vulnerable: The afflictions known as housemaid's knee and tennis elbow are familiar examples.

While arthritic ailments come in many forms, even a brief rundown of the major types reveals an obvious fact: Joint pain can mean any number of things. An aching knee might arise from a simple sprain, or from bursitis, osteoarthritis, gout, or a related disease. It could stem from a wear-and-tear process or be an indication of a more generalized disease. Some patients experience joint pain that defies quick analysis. For example, it may take weeks or months to make a firm diagnosis of rheumatoid arthritis. Complicating the picture is the fact that systemic lupus can occasionally be confused with rheumatoid arthritis. The joint involvement in these diseases may be virtually identical and, until recently, laboratory tests could not be relied on to distinguish between them. Nowadays, improved laboratory tests make an accurate diagnosis more likely.

Beyond diagnosis, the treatment for a specific disease may be different for different people. One arthritis patient may respond well to a particular drug, while another with the same illness may gain only marginal relief or experience intolerable side effects. In short, diagnosis and treatment of arthritic diseases can be a complicated process, often requiring patience and cooperation on the part of the patient.

In contrast, unproved or irrational remedies are usually hawked as panaceas to all comers. Such answers to pain and crippling are available to everyone willing to spend the money to try a convenient bottle, the latest fad in diet books, or a publicized clinic offering a secret or a miraculous cure. It sometimes seems as though every type of offbeat treatment has been promoted for arthritis. The gimmicks run the gamut from copper bracelets and "immune" milk to mechanical contraptions, radioactive pads, and potent drugs. And arthritis sufferers are apparently good customers for such items. Mailing lists of arthritics are used over and over. Once patients order something from an advertiser, they're likely to get a stream of mail for a whole grab bag of products.

Today, the emphasis in arthritis promotions is shifting—heavier on diet fads and unproved drugs, lighter on contraptions. For many years, mechanical devices and oddball gimmicks were a prime staple of arthritis quackery. For $9.95 you could order the *Miracle Health Relaxer,* which promised relief for both arthritis and constipation. A *Vryllium Tube* cost you a bit more; it contained two cents worth of salt and sold for $250. By contrast, the *Vivicosmic Disk* was a bargain—only $5 for a piece of cement. Among the most popular devices were vibrators. One model for arthritics came with five attachments, including one guaranteed to banish dandruff. And there was the *Pulse-A-Rhythm* vibrating mattress, until the U.S. Food and Drug Administration seized the product, calling it ineffective and dangerous for those it was touted to help.

For a while, radiation was in. Arthritis victims could pay for the privilege of sitting in an abandoned uranium mine to absorb the "healing radiations." If they were too poor or too crippled to take advantage of this sovereign remedy, they could still buy mitts or pads supposedly containing low-grade radioactive ore. A typical one, the *Marvpad,* cost $30 and was filled with gravel. Most such gimmicks have now faded from the market, according to the Arthritis Foundation. And federal legislation passed in 1976 to regulate the marketing of medical devices should help prevent new examples from surfacing. Moreover, there's now a much more respectable source of income than yesterday's sleazy gadgets. Arthritis-cure promoters have rediscovered nutrition.

Worthless diet cures have always been a part of arthritis mythology. If the magic nutrient wasn't cod liver oil, it might have been alfalfa, or pokeberries, or *Honegar*—the mixture concocted by the late D. C. Jarvis, M.D., out of honey and vinegar plus a bit of iodine and kelp. However, in recent years there has been a virtual bandwagon of public interest in many aspects of nutrition, including claims of attaining "super health" at the dinner table. Arthritis-cure promoters have been quick to join the parade, and several arthritis diet books have flourished.

When *The Arthritic's Cookbook* sold well, out came a sequel, *New Hope for the Arthritic* (same diet). If your appetite was unsatisfied but your joints still ached, you could turn to another heavily advertised candidate, *A Doctor's* Proven *New Home Cure for Arthritis.* No relief? Perhaps *There* Is *a Cure for Arthritis* would hit on the right menu. Eventually, the Arthritis Foundation, which maintains a list of books *not* recommended for arthritics (see pages 68–69) added a special section for the growing assortment of diet cure-alls.

The truth is that there's no scientific evidence that any food or vitamin has anything to do with causing or curing arthritis. "The proper diet for someone with arthritis," advises the Arthritis Foundation, "is a normal, well-balanced, nourishing diet—the same things people without arthritis should eat. The one exception is with gouty arthritis. Certain foods—primarily organ meats such as liver and kidneys—may increase uric acid levels in the blood and should be avoided." Some arthritis victims who are overweight may need a reducing diet to ease the burden on weight-bearing joints. But, otherwise, diet regimens touted for arthritis are about as useful as the *Pulse-A-Rhythm* mattress or the *Vivicosmic Disk.*

Meanwhile, some over-the-counter drug marketers are not averse to cashing in on the arthritis patient's discomfort. Plain aspirin is the most effective OTC drug for arthritis. And many arthritis patients buy lots of it. A person with active rheumatoid arthritis who is being treated with aspirin may have to take as many as fifteen 5-grain tablets daily. Plain aspirin is relatively cheap. But over a period of months and years, the nickels and dimes mount up. And they mount up a lot faster if the patient can be persuaded through exposure to constant advertising to buy a more expensive OTC product containing aspirin.

The makers of *Anacin,* for example, have noted in their advertising that "the pain medication doctors prescribe most for arthritis also has a most effective anti-inflammatory action. What you should know is that this same medication is in today's *Anacin* tablets." The medication, of course, is aspirin—at several times the price of plain aspirin tablets. And it's the same ingredient in *Arthritis Pain Formula, Arthritis Strength Bufferin,* and *Ascriptin.* The tablet size is a bit larger, and there is antacid added. But the products are essentially expensive forms of aspirin. You pay for the tinsel.

An expert advisory panel that reviewed OTC pain relievers for the Food and Drug Administration recommended in 1977 that the agency prohibit all claims for arthritis relief in the labeling or name of aspirin products. "Consumers who self-treat with an OTC pain reliever for these [arthritic] diseases, without first seeking medical attention, may be risking irreversible damage to joints and other tissues," the FDA panel said. Consumers Union's medical consultants agree emphatically with that statement.

Liniments, ointments, and body rubs are also heavily

promoted for relief of aches and pains from arthritis. These OTC products depend on one or more skin irritants for their effect—usually methyl salicylate (oil of wintergreen) and various combinations of others. Application of these external analgesics tends to increase blood flow in the upper layers of the skin, resulting in a slight reddening of the skin as well as a sensation of warmth. The mild increase in skin temperature may provide brief symptomatic relief. However, CU's medical consultants warn against indiscriminate use of external analgesics with high methyl salicylate content. Some products, such as *Ben-Gay Extra Strength Balm, Exocaine,* and *Panalgesic,* have concentrations of 30 percent or more. The substance can be absorbed through the skin, and excessive amounts can result in poisoning. Note that absorption would be speeded up if the drug were applied to mucous membranes or to areas where the skin is cut or inflamed. Preparations containing methyl salicylate should never be used for children. Nor should any liniment be used in conjunction with a heating pad. Severe burns with blistering may result.

Over the years, any number of doctors have publicized offbeat remedies or therapies for arthritis. If the regimens later proved to be ineffective, they often fell by the wayside. But not always. The physician's faith in the remedy—or faith in its money-making potential—could help to generate enough publicity to keep it alive. And any remedy, no matter how controversial, can seem inviting to an arthritis victim in chronic pain.

Among the holdovers still attracting attention is dimethyl sulfoxide, or DMSO. First publicized in the early 1960s, DMSO was touted as a possible treatment for various ailments, including musculoskeletal injuries and some arthritic diseases. In 1978 the FDA approved its use for interstitial cystitis, a bladder disorder. Although this was the first time DMSO had been approved in the United States for human beings, it had been sanctioned as a veterinary drug in 1970, which, in effect, made it generally available for additional unauthorized use.

In 1974 the National Academy of Sciences/National Research Council called for studies of DMSO in several disorders. In addition to its evaluation in interstitial cystitis, DMSO was tested on patients with scleroderma, an uncommon connective tissue disease primarily affecting the skin, esophagus, lung, kidneys, and, at times, the joints as well. It failed to be of help. To date, the possible effectiveness of DMSO in any long-term treatment of rheumatic disease has not been established. Nevertheless, campaigns similar to those mounted for the cancer nostrum Laetrile (see Chapter Two) have won legalization for uses of DMSO in Oregon (1977) and Florida (1978) that are not allowed on the federal level. And several clinics in Mexico claim to treat arthritis patients with DMSO (however, some drugs brought back to the United States from such clinics have contained potent ingredients other than DMSO).

Meanwhile, alleged breakthroughs in arthritis treatment are heralded from time to time in newspapers and magazines. Three typical "cures" that received wide publicity in the last few years were each radically different from one another. In one, arthritis was reported to be an allergic disease that could be alleviated by a starvation diet. In another, some five hundred arthritis patients were said to have improved dramatically after treatment with a flu vaccine. In a third, arthritis patients were supposedly helped by taking tablets derived from yucca plants. Both the vaccine and the yucca treatments were advocated by the same physicians, Bernard A. Bellew and Robert Bingham of Desert Hot Springs, California. When arthritis specialists associated with the Arthritis Foundation investigated the reports, they could find no scientific evidence to back up the claims. No controlled trials of the various therapies had been conducted, and the studies the specialists reviewed were inadequate to support any claimed benefit.

Any physician knows how to relieve severe arthritic pain. Cortisone and similar steroid drugs can provide dramatic reduction of pain and inflammation in a matter of hours or days. But daily use of steroids for prolonged periods can cause serious side effects, particularly at high dosage levels. These effects can sometimes be more severe than the arthritis, and even life-threatening. Accordingly, while steroids and other potent drugs still have a valuable place in arthritis treatment, their use is commonly reserved for specific situations where the benefits outweigh the risks.

In recent decades, however, a number of physicians have gained notoriety and wealth by dispensing large quantities of steroid concoctions and other potentially dangerous drugs. Lured by the hope of a cure, thousands of patients have traveled to clinics in Canada, the Dominican Republic, or Mexico to obtain such drugs as Liefcort, Rheumatril, or unnamed "secret" remedies.

The father of Liefcort was the late Robert E. Liefmann, M.D., who fled the United States for Canada in 1957 to avoid prosecution for distributing a purported baldness cure. He first attracted wide public attention in May 1962, when *Look* magazine ran an article about his creation of Liefcort. Initially described as a home-brewed hormone remedy, Liefcort turned out on analysis to be a combination of three well-known drugs—prednisone (a steroid), testosterone (a male hormone), and estradiol (a female hormone). The FDA characterized it as "an irrational mixture of potent ingredients." In an official statement, the FDA noted: "We believe that Liefcort is dangerous to any person who uses it, even when used under medical supervision."

Despite legal run-ins with Canadian authorities, Liefmann managed to continue operating a clinic in Montreal for several years and to dispense Liefcort to thousands of patients. American arthritis patients streamed across the border to pay $9 an ounce for it. The price later jumped to $30 an ounce, with a minimum purchase of $180. In 1969 Liefmann was convicted on sixteen counts of violating Canada's Food and Drugs Act and was fined $2,400. He died in 1972 with the case still under appeal. The formula he concocted lives on, however.

At least two organizations in the United States promote the Liefmann treatment method under such names as "Balanced Hormone Therapy" and "Balanced Hormone Treatment for Arthritics." One is the Arthritis Medical Information Society—originally called the Arthritis Medical Center—in New York City. It has a chapter in Hollywood, Florida, as well. Another is an association called M.A.R.T.A., which is based in Charleston, South Carolina. Both organizations have been associated with Elizabeth R. Daley, M.D., a long-time friend of Liefmann's.

The Liefmann concoction also survives in Santo Domingo, Dominican Republic, where a version of it goes under the name of Rheumatril. It's dispensed at a clinic headed by William Jana, M.D., an associate of Liefmann's widow. Similarly potent and dangerous drugs are dispensed for take-out customers at three notorious clinics in Mexico. One is operated by Luis Carrillo, M.D., in Mexicali. Another is run by Ernesto Chavarria, M.D., in Piedras Negras. A third is located in Juarez. Two of the clinics have been in business for years, and all reportedly do a brisk trade. Various medical sources have reported serious adverse reactions and a number of deaths among patients who visited the Liefmann clinic in Canada or the Mexicali clinic. CU is unaware of comparable reports concerning the other clinics, but we would expect the toll in serious drug-induced illness to be similar at these clinics.

Arthritis-cure promoters know the importance of publicity and are often skillful at using the media to advantage. Liefcort became an overnight success on the strength of one magazine story. But arthritis can be a money-maker for the press as well. A potential market of almost 32 million sufferers makes arthritis a prime topic for publications that trade in sensationalism. National weekly tabloids like the *National Enquirer* and the *Midnight Globe* run numerous stories

Health Quackery

on the subject—often with banner headlines on page one.

Offbeat treatment schemes get almost automatic coverage. But if quacks happen to lie low for a few months, the tabloids are capable of turning the merest hint of a research development into a breakthrough seemingly worthy of a Nobel Prize. A brief research report about preliminary results of a drug trial with fourteen patients came out this way in the *National Enquirer:* Page one carried the banner headline, "ARTHRITIS CURE." The headline of the story stated, "Top Medical University Breakthrough for 50 Million Americans—Arthritis Cure." The story told of the drug's "remarkable success" with some 540 patients— 526 more than reported—and the prospect of giving "quick relief to the 50 million Americans . . . who suffer from arthritis." Apparently, besides aiding 526 phantom patients, the drug is potent enough to cure arthritis in some 18 million Americans who don't even have any symptoms of the disease.

The story is typical of the reporting on arthritis that appears in the national tabloids and sometimes in other publications as well. *Prevention* magazine, for example, often publishes enthusiastic articles promoting various vitamin and mineral supplements as arthritis remedies. According to the Arthritis Foundation, sensationalized accounts of miraculous remedies or purported cures represent a major problem for the victims of arthritis. "They first hear about these dubious treatments from a paper with a circulation of millions sold mostly in supermarkets," Charles Bennett, the foundation's education director, has noted. "In their desperate search for relief, they will try anything, no matter how crazy it may sound, no matter how much it may cost."

Although there is still no cure, arthritis is no longer the hopeless disease it once was. Over the last generation, advances in therapy have greatly improved the prospects for arthritis victims. With early diagnosis and treatment, many patients can now avoid disability and lead relatively normal lives.

Current therapy takes several forms, including medication, exercise, and other physical measures. In cases of severe joint damage, surgery may be utilized. Individual treatment varies widely, depending on the type of arthritis, its severity, and the patient's response to therapy. Treatment can even differ for the same disease. Whatever the ailment, though, the most important step in the treatment process is proper diagnosis.

About one out of every six visits to a family physician or internist is for problems involving muscles, joints, tendons, or ligaments. Many such complaints arise from localized muscle pain or some other self-limited symptom that will clear up in a few days even without treatment. All that may be needed is rest and a mild pain medication. But claims for unproved or quack arthritis remedies are frequently based on "successful" treatment of just such ailments.

If pain in one or more joints persists for a week or two, or recurs over a period of weeks, a physician should be consulted. Gonorrhea, gout, rheumatoid arthritis, and occasionally osteoarthritis may begin as an acute inflammatory arthritis, with redness, heat, pain, and swelling of the involved joint. Such dramatic symp-

57

toms usually prompt the victim to seek immediate medical attention. More often, though, arthritis symptoms come on gradually. The symptoms may appear for a few days and go away, then come back stronger and disappear again. There may be weeks or months between goings and comings, but gradually the disease reappears at shorter intervals until it becomes a daily problem that is more difficult to ignore.

Flare-ups and remissions are common in rheumatoid arthritis, ankylosing spondylitis (arthritis of the spine), and other inflammatory arthritic diseases. Consequently, any recurring joint symptoms should be checked with a doctor, no matter how mild or "temporary" they might appear at first. Physical examination, X rays, and specific laboratory tests can help distinguish arthritis from less serious ailments and differentiate one type of arthritis from another. Sometimes examination of the joint fluid is also necessary. The sooner treatment begins, the greater the likelihood of avoiding permanent joint damage.

Medication is the first line of defense against arthritis. The immediate goal of drug therapy is to reduce inflammation and pain. Ultimately, the objective is to preserve joint function. The reduction in pain and swelling helps the patient to maintain joint mobility, which might otherwise not be possible. The anti-inflammatory effect also serves to minimize or prevent joint damage.

The most frequently prescribed drug for arthritis is aspirin. Its familiarity as a household remedy for minor aches and pains often makes people doubt that aspirin can work effectively against serious forms of arthritis.

But it does. In large doses, commonly ten to fifteen 5-grain tablets daily, aspirin is as effective in suppressing joint inflammation as the newer and costlier drugs noted below. As such, it's often the first choice in treatment. Although aspirin is the mainstay for a majority of arthritis patients, it is not a perfect drug. People vary in their tolerance for aspirin, and some cannot take it at all. Large doses may cause stomach irritation and gastrointestinal bleeding, which can be mild or severe. Other common side effects include ringing in the ears and temporary hearing loss. To control such effects, physicians may reduce the dosage, prescribe aspirin combined with antacid or enteric-coated aspirin, or try other salicylate drugs similar to aspirin, such as choline salicylate or sodium salicylate. (Acetaminophen, a common aspirin substitute for minor aches and pains, is not effective against inflammation.)

Some patients, however, may not get adequate relief from aspirin or other salicylates. Nor are these drugs effective in all arthritic disorders. In such instances, other drugs are used. In the treatment of acute gout, for example, aspirin has no place, and physicians may prescribe another anti-inflammatory agent or colchicine, a medication used for decades in the treatment of acute gout. In infectious types of arthritis, the early use of antibiotics can spell the difference between cure and a chronically stiff, deformed joint. With osteoarthritis and rheumatoid arthritis, however, finding the right drug can be a process of trial and error. Generally, the safest drugs that are likely to be of benefit are tried first. Several drugs may be evaluated, in varying dosages, until the best one is found.

A drug sometimes used in place of aspirin is indomethacin. Introduced in 1965 under the brand name Indocin, its side effects include not only stomach irritation (as is common with aspirin), but also headache, which may be severe. Nevertheless, about 25 percent of patients with rheumatoid arthritis show good or excellent improvement with indomethacin, so the drug may be tried when aspirin is ineffective or poorly tolerated. Clinical experience suggests that indomethacin may also be helpful in arthritis of the cervical spine, gout, psoriatic arthritis, and osteoarthritis, particularly osteoarthritis of the hip.

Since 1974, five new drugs have been introduced that offer alternatives for individualized therapy. The first was ibuprofen (Motrin), soon followed by naproxen (Naprosyn), fenoprofen (Nalfon), tolmetin (Tolectin), and, most recently, sulindac (Clinoril). In appropriate dosages, the drugs are comparable to aspirin in anti-inflammatory effect, and for some patients their side effects seem milder than those from high doses of aspirin. All are far more expensive than aspirin.

While none of the newer drugs represents a breakthrough, these agents provide much more flexibility in treatment than had been previously possible. Since individual patients may respond better to one drug than to another, the availability of several choices increases the chances of finding an optimum regimen for more patients—particularly those who don't do well on aspirin.

Aspirin, indomethacin, and the five new agents are considered the safest drugs for long-term treatment, and physicians commonly turn to them first. If a patient doesn't respond adequately, however, there are others that may be used. All involve a greater risk of serious side effects than the initial group of drugs. But they can be helpful to patients who might not otherwise obtain relief.

Phenylbutazone was introduced in 1949 for treating rheumatoid arthritis and related disorders. It is available generically and under various brand names, including Azolid and Butazolidin. It is an effective anti-inflammatory agent, but its potential side effects on the kidneys, stomach, and bone marrow usually limit it to short-term use. At times, though, it is used for extended therapy under close medical supervision, which includes periodic blood counts and urinalyses. Some clinicians believe it to be especially effective for spinal arthritis. A chemically related drug, oxyphenbutazone (Tandearil), exhibits similar effects.

Drugs known as antimalarials are sometimes used for rheumatoid arthritis and systemic lupus erythematosus, as well as for the prevention of malaria. Derived from quinine, antimalarials may help to reduce symptoms when prescribed in limited doses over a long period of time. Because these drugs can produce serious side effects, especially in the eye, their use must be carefully monitored. Two commonly used antimalarials are chloroquine and hydroxychloroquine; both are generic drugs.

Among the oldest compounds used to treat rheumatoid arthritis are gold salts. For many years there was uncertainty about how well gold worked in reducing the severity of inflammation. But recent studies have established its effectiveness in selected cases of rheumatoid arthritis that don't respond to other treatment. It usually takes six to twelve weeks to find out whether gold therapy benefits a patient. Treatment is started with weekly administration, and patients are watched carefully for side effects, which may include skin rash, bone marrow depression, and kidney damage. Gold salts have to be given by injection and require periodic blood counts and urinalyses, which can make for a costly program.

There is a potential substitute for gold treatment in the drug penicillamine (Cuprimine, Depen), which was approved by the Food and Drug Administration in 1978 for use in rheumatoid arthritis. Patients who don't respond to gold treatment or can't tolerate it may be candidates for penicillamine. Although chemically related to penicillin, penicillamine is not an antibiotic. It has been used successfully for more than twenty years to treat Wilson's disease, a disorder of copper metabolism, which affects the liver and brain. Its efficacy in rheumatoid arthritis is also well established. The problem is its toxicity. The most common side effect is skin rash, but serious blood and kidney disorders can also occur, sometimes very quickly, making it imperative to stop the drug immediately. Approximately two-thirds of patients experience moderate to severe side effects. Clinical trials indicate that penicillamine is at least as effective as gold therapy in severe rheumatoid arthritis. Like gold, it is very slow-acting and can take months to produce beneficial effects. Several additional months may be required to adjust the dosage properly. Because of its toxicity, the drug is generally reserved for severe rheumatoid arthritis that does not respond to other therapy.

Experimental drugs now under study for arthritis include agents that suppress the body's immune system, its natural defense against foreign organisms. Research indicates that cells that normally protect the body may actually contribute to the inflammatory process in some forms of arthritis. Hence, certain immunosuppressive drugs used for cancer treatment or for organ transplantation are being tried, on a limited basis, for severe rheumatoid arthritis and lupus. Among the agents being evaluated in the United States are azathioprine and cyclophosphamide. Since such drugs can be highly toxic, their use is commonly limited to severe and unresponsive cases.

Cortisone-related steroids, such as prednisone, are another class of drugs that must be used with caution. As noted earlier in the chapter, steroids are the most potent anti-inflammatory drugs available and can provide dramatic relief of pain and swelling in inflamed joints. However, their numerous side effects limit their usefulness in prolonged therapy. Unlike gold salts and penicillamine, which can be well tolerated by some patients for years, steroids eventually produce serious side effects in all patients during extended therapy, unless given in very low dosage. Accordingly, in certain cases when oral steroids are the only alternative, they are generally used in the smallest amounts that will improve symptoms—sometimes on an every-other-day basis. Direct injection of steroids into a particularly painful joint is still a common method of providing relief, however, and is relatively free of hazard if used infrequently.

While medication is the cornerstone of arthritis treatment, physical measures are also important. Part of the goal is to achieve a proper balance between rest and exercise. During a flare-up, rest can be as important as medication. Complete body rest, usually in bed, helps to reduce inflammation. Exercise must be kept to a minimum to prevent further damage to affected joints. Heat treatment, such as hot soaks, baths, and showers, are commonly prescribed to relieve pain and stiffness. Occasionally, a patient will respond better to cold packs around an acutely inflamed joint than to heat. Whirlpool baths or other forms of hydrotherapy may also be advised for some patients. Individual joints are sometimes rested in removable, lightweight splints. That helps lessen inflammation and keeps the joint in a normal-use position, protecting it against muscle flexion deformities (contractures) that might lead to permanent disfigurement. Splints can also be used to help straighten out a joint that has become fixed in a flexed position. The splints are usually adjusted every few days to move the joint toward the desired position.

Once inflammation and pain subside, more emphasis is placed on exercise. For arthritis patients, exercise does not mean engaging in athletics or similarly strenuous activities. It involves putting joints gently through their full range of motion every day. This helps maintain normal joint movement and aids in strengthening muscles that may have been weakened by inactivity. As joint function improves, the exercises may be done against slight resistance, provided there is no pain. Generally, each patient requires an individually prescribed program of exercises. Occupational therapy can help patients master the tasks of everyday living despite painful disabilities.

If an appropriate program of rest and exercise is followed faithfully, it serves not only to prevent deformities but also to help correct those that might have developed. One problem, however, is that some patients who feel better forgo their exercises and even medication. The result may be an earlier or more severe return of symptoms than might otherwise have occurred. Until recent years, severe arthritic damage to a joint usually meant chronic pain and permanent disability. Once the damage was done, it was irreversible. For many patients, however, that's no longer true. Since the early 1960s, when the first successful total hip-joint replacement was performed, numerous surgical techniques have been developed to undo the crippling effects of arthritis. Total hip replacement represents one of the major advances in orthopedic surgery of the past century. Introduced in England by John Charnley, M.D., the procedure utilized a joint made of metal and plastic parts secured in place with bone cement. The development of a fully artificial joint launched a successful collaboration between surgeons and engineers to overcome orthopedic problems that were once considered hopeless.

The knowledge gained in hip surgery has since fostered many advances in the replacement of other joints. The knee joint—a common site of arthritic damage—can now be replaced with artificial components.

And research is in progress on similar operations for the hand, wrist, elbow, ankle, and shoulder. Complications or failure can occur with any of the operations, and not every patient with a severe disability is a candidate for joint replacement. For many patients, though, the operations can relieve pain, correct deformities, and improve joint function.

Other surgical techniques besides joint replacement have also been developed for arthritic problems. Removal of diseased tissue in the joint capsule may relieve pain for a period of years. Bow leg or knock knee caused by joint erosion may be corrected by an osteotomy, which realigns the bone by removing from it a small, wedge-shaped section. An unstable joint may be fused to stiffen the bone, usually to relieve pain and correct deformity. A joint may also be reconstructed, sometimes using similar tissue from another part of the body.

To a large extent, the success of joint surgery depends on the patient's willingness to participate actively in a lengthy postoperative therapy program. Appropriate exercise is essential to gain function and strength in the reconstructed parts. Without such effort, the best surgical procedures may fail.

When people first seek medical help for arthritis symptoms, they ordinarily turn to an internist or family physician. When diagnosis and treatment of the more serious forms of arthritis require specialized knowledge, the patients may be referred to a rheumatologist, a specialist in arthritic diseases. The Arthritis Foundation, a national voluntary health organization that provides information and other assistance to arthritis victims, can supply the names of qualified rheumatologists in your area. The foundation has seventy-three local chapters in major American cities. If you can't locate the chapter serving your area, write to the foundation at Lenox P.O. Box 18888, Atlanta, Georgia 30326.

A Guide to Books on Arthritis

Because of the large potential readership, books on arthritis are constantly being published. To help arthritis patients separate the good from the bad, the Arthritis Foundation regularly reviews such books for medical accuracy and scientific validity. Since its book list is long and includes a number of titles now out of print, only a partial selection appears below. For information about other books on arthritis and related diseases, consult any of the foundation's local chapters.

The following books provide reliable and helpful information about arthritis, according to the Arthritis Foundation.

Arthritis—Complete, Up-to-Date Facts for Patients and Their Families by Sheldon P. Blau, M.D., and Dodi Schultz. (Doubleday & Co., Inc., Garden City, N.Y.) 1974. $5.95

Arthritis: A Comprehensive Guide by James F. Fries, M.D. (Addison-Wesley Publishing Co., Reading, Mass., and Menlo Park, Ca.) 1979. $11.95; paperback, $6.95

The Arthritis Handbook—A Patient's Manual on Arthritis, Rheumatism and Gout by Darrell C. Crain, M.D. (Arco Publishing, New York) 2nd edition, revised 1971. $6.50

Beyond the Copper Bracelet: What You Should Know About Arthritis by Louis A. Healey, M.D., Kenneth R. Wilske, M.D., and Bob Hansen. (Charles Press, Bowie, Md.) 2nd edition, 1977. $5.95

Living With Your Arthritis edited by Alan M. Rosenberg, M.D. (Arco Publishing, New York) 1979. $8.95; paperback, $3.95

Lupus: The Body Against Itself by Sheldon P. Blau, M.D., and Dodi Schultz. (Doubleday & Co., Inc., Garden City, N.Y.) 1977. $5.95

The Truth About Arthritis Care by John J. Calabro, M.D., and John Wykert. (David McKay Co., Inc., New York) 1971. $7.95

Understanding Arthritis and Rheumatism: A Complete Guide to the Problems and Treatment by Malcolm I. V. Jayson, M.D., and Allan St. J. Dixon, M.D. (Pantheon Books, New York) 1975. $7.95; Dell paperback, 1976, $1.75

You Asked About Rheumatoid Arthritis by Harold Speers Robinson, M.D. (Douglas & McIntyre, Vancouver) 1978. $5.95

The following books *do not* meet the Arthritis Foundation's criteria for medical accuracy and scientific validity.

The Arthritic's Cookbook by Colin M. Dong, M.D., and Jane Banks

Arthritis Can Be Cured—A Layman's Guide by Bernard Aschner, M.D.

Arthritis, Nutrition and Natural Therapy by Carlson Wade

Bees Don't Get Arthritis by Fred Malone

A Doctor's *Proven* New Home Cure for Arthritis by Giraud W. Campbell, D.O., and R. Stone

The Miraculous Holistic Balanced Treatment for Arthritis Diseases by Henry B. Rothblatt, J.D., LL.M., Donna Pinorsky, R.N., and Michael Brodsky

New Hope for the Arthritic by Colin M. Dong, M.D., and Jane Banks

The Nightshades and Health by Norman Franklin Childers and Gerard M. Russo

Pain-Free Arthritis by Dvera Berson with Sander Roy

There *Is* a Cure for Arthritis by Paavo O. Airola

You Can Stay Well and **Let's Get Well** by Adelle Davis, M.S.

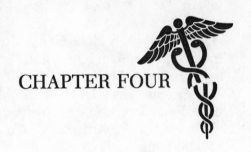

CHAPTER FOUR

Low Blood Sugar: Fiction and Fact

Some afflictions, such as arthritis and cancer, are so widespread and so painful that they become a fertile field for ingenious promoters of purported cures. Working the other side of the street are those who exploit people with a variety of general symptoms by fitting them all neatly into a single diagnostic category. Hypoglycemia—or low blood sugar, as it is commonly called —is just such a grab bag.

Hypoglycemia is a real enough disorder, although relatively uncommon. However, it has also become the easy catchall for a collection of ill-defined symptoms. As a result, the questionable practices of a small minority of doctors account for far more "victims" of hypoglycemia than do valid medical indications. A few doctors have found it convenient—and profitable—to label patients hypoglycemic, usually without laboratory evidence to substantiate the diagnosis. And even when these doctors do run proper diagnostic tests, they misinterpret—or ignore—the laboratory evidence. And some food faddists have also latched onto hypoglycemia as a condition resulting from faulty diet and poor nutrition.

A world of fiction has been created about hypoglycemia. For a variety of reasons, many people at times experience fatigue, insomnia, irritability, faintness, depression, and a host of other burdensome complaints. Few such people suffer from low blood sugar. Low blood sugar in and of itself—and unrelated to a specific physical disorder—is seldom responsible for such complaints. Nevertheless, a small number of physicians, nutritionists, and self-styled "health" publications would have people believe that many of those emotional disorders and vague feelings of being unwell result from low blood sugar.

Despite the relative infrequency of documented hypoglycemia, it has received widespread publicity in books and magazines. For example, in its April 1979 issue, *Prevention* magazine claimed that "an estimated 50 million" Americans suffer from hypoglycemia. From where does all this publicity come?

For years, the leading drumbeater has been the Hypoglycemia Foundation, Inc., a low-budget, tax-exempt organization that operated until recently from the suburban New York apartment of one of its officers. Its stated goal has been "to put recognition and treatment of hypoglycemia on a par with diabetes" and to alert physicians to hypoglycemia "and indoctrinate them in its proper treatment." Its publication "Delinquent Glands Not Juvenile Delinquents" suggests that "a goodly percentage of juvenile delinquents would become happily well adjusted individuals if their hypoglycemia were recognized and treated." Another pamphlet advises that "controlling hypoglycemia is frequently relatively simple, and that such control could do much to prevent diabetes and to reduce alcoholism and drug addiction"; it would also combat "mental retardation, chronic fatigue, asthma, allergies, and many other serious problems."

People apparently hear of the foundation by word of mouth, in the pages of *Prevention,* or through a handful of widely sold books. One of these, *Goodbye Allergies,* has sold more than fifty thousand copies. Its author, Tom R. Blaine, an Oklahoma judge, now retired, describes himself as a "cured" hypoglycemic. His book portrays hypoglycemia as something of a modern-day black plague and attributes many of the world's problems to low blood sugar.

A foundation official, Marilyn Light, who learned about hypoglycemia from Blaine's book and who claims to have been restored to full health by the diet and treatment he described, told Consumers Union in 1971 that about three hundred physicians in forty-two states and the District of Columbia were registered with the Hypoglycemia Foundation. Marilyn Light said most of those physicians had an average case load of two hundred fifty "hypoglycemia" patients. (A doctor in Salt Lake City was said to be treating five hundred people.) *Prevention* claims that some two thousand doctors are currently "affiliated" with the foundation.

The fountainhead of much of the erroneous information disseminated by the Hypoglycemia Foundation and its physician-allies is the teachings of the late John Tintera, M.D., of Yonkers, New York. Tintera's involvement with hypoglycemia followed publication in 1951 of *Body, Mind and Sugar,* by E. M. Abrahamson, M.D., and A. W. Pezet. The book, which has been frequently reprinted, attributed to low blood sugar a variety of mental and physical disorders supposedly affecting millions of Americans. This same condition, the authors claimed, was responsible "for the moral breakdown that underlies all delinquency and crime." The authors conceded that their views were not accepted by the medical profession, but that this was "largely because most doctors have not yet had time to read the literature."

In a series of medical journal articles published in the late 1950s and early 1960s, Tintera went beyond Abrahamson's claims. Tintera recommended periodic injections of adrenal cortical extract (a relatively weak extract of hog and beef adrenals), generally referred to as ACE. These injections, of course, involved considerable expense to the patient.

Used initially as a treatment for chronic Addison's disease (a serious disorder due to atrophy of the adrenal glands), ACE was already an obsolete drug when it was first touted for alleged victims of hypoglycemia. The use of ACE in treating hypoglycemia was based on the notion that low blood sugar is always caused by inadequate secretion of certain hormones by the adrenal glands. The adrenals are best known for the manner in which they bring a person to full alertness and energy in a crisis, but they also help to stabilize the level of blood sugar. Low blood sugar was said to be associated with "tired" or "worn out" adrenal glands, and injections of ACE were supposed to increase the blood sugar level. Actually, there is no evidence that adrenal insufficiency plays any role in functional hypoglycemia, the most common form of the ailment (see page 78.) Nor is there any evidence that ACE has a place in the treatment of hypoglycemia—or, for that matter in the treatment of *any* disease.

In 1958 Tintera presented some of his views in a series of articles in *Woman's Day* magazine, causing his peers in the Westchester County (New York) Medical Society to call him to appear before it. Tintera was censured by the society for publishing in a lay magazine an article on endocrinology, a subject in which he allegedly had no formal postgraduate medical training. Some time later, the society received a complaint from a young university professor who claimed that Tintera had given him weekly injections of ACE for seven months. Tintera reportedly told the young man that he would need the injections for the rest of his life. After having spent hundreds of dollars on ACE, the young man entered a hospital for a series of tests, which revealed no abnormalities. In 1967 the Westchester County Medical Society advised Tintera to abandon his treatment for hypoglycemia. But there is nothing to suggest that Tintera did abandon his particular brand of medicine prior to his death in 1969.

Aside from the mild rebuke to Tintera, CU found little evidence until 1973 that organized medicine was trying to crack down on physicians who administered ACE for hypoglycemia. The fictions flourishing around this fad ailment and its treatment moved CU to set the record straight in a July 1971 article in CONSUMER REPORTS. It was not until January 1973, however, that the medical establishment finally saw fit to follow suit. Three prominent organizations of physicians and scientists—the American Diabetes Association, the American Medical Association, and the Endocrine Society—issued a joint statement echoing the CU position. The organizations stated that "the majority of people" with symptoms of sweating, shakiness, trembling, anxiety, fast heart action, headache, hunger sensations, brief feelings of weakness, and, occasionally, seizures and coma "do not have hypoglycemia." The organizations pointed out that many patients with symptoms of this kind may be suffering from anxiety reactions.

Reviewing the medical facts of the disorder, these organizations voiced the same judgment about ACE that Consumers Union had expressed in CONSUMER REPORTS two years earlier. Their joint statement said, in dismissing ACE, that "there is no known medical use for it." The statement stressed that administration of ACE "is not an appropriate treatment for any cause of hypoglycemia." CU welcomed the statement and expressed the hope that it might signal some stirring within the medical profession to take effective action against doctors who persisted in treating their patients with ACE. According to CU's medical consultants, if some of these patients felt better, their improvement was probably due less to ACE than to the fact that their physician was taking their complaints seriously and appeared to be trying to help them.

Eventually, the U.S. Food and Drug Administration ordered ACE off the market. Said the agency in 1977: "There is no evidence it is effective in treating burns, low blood sugar, alcohol or drug addiction, or any other disease. In the treatment of Addison's disease, the drug is too weak to be effective."

With the demise of ACE, advocates of the notion that low blood sugar is a national plague have rallied around other nostrums. Often these include a host of nutritional supplements, such as vitamins, minerals, brewer's yeast, and the like. In short, the hypoglycemia fiction is still alive and thriving in the pages of various health-fad books and magazines.

But what are the facts about hypoglycemia? *Hypo* (low) *glycemia* (sugar in the blood) is not a disease. Nor is it a syndrome unless a particular complex of symptoms is accompanied by a biochemical abnormality, established by a laboratory test. Nor is it a constant condition; almost invariably, attacks are intermittent, with perfectly normal intervals between episodes.

The level of sugar in the blood is maintained within certain limits by the opposing actions of different physiological forces. Blood sugar is increased by eating foods containing sugar or starches or by the release of sugar stored in the liver in the form of a complex carbohydrate, glycogen. Two potent hormones that cause the liver to release sugar are glucagon (made in the pancreas) and adrenaline (made in the adrenal glands). Counteracting these hormones is insulin, another hormone, manufactured in and released by the pancreas. Insulin facilitates the utilization of blood sugar by the various cells of the body, which then transform the sugar into energy. The usual stimulus to the release of insulin is an increase in blood sugar level.

When the blood sugar falls in rapid fashion to a significantly subnormal level, a surge of adrenaline is released from the adrenal glands as the body attempts to restore the low blood sugar to a normal level. Adrenaline causes glycogen, stored in the liver, to break down and release sugar into the bloodstream, thereby restoring the blood sugar to normal levels. In the process, the rapid release of adrenaline also affects the heart and the nervous system, causing such symptoms as trembling, sweating, palpitations, nervousness, and headache.

A second variety of hypoglycemic symptoms is due to the direct effect of the low blood sugar itself on the functioning of the central nervous system. These usually occur at a blood sugar level lower than the level that triggers the adrenaline-release symptoms. As the blood sugar level continues to fall, the more severe symptoms occur. They include mental aberrations, personality changes, bizarre behavior, and even temporary amnesia. These abnormalities of central nervous system functioning tend to follow a repetitive pattern, each episode being characterized by the same set of behavioral abnormalities.

Most hypoglycemic episodes can be dramatically relieved by the ingestion or injection of glucose (sugar) or by an injection of glucagon. Severe hypoglycemic reactions may require the use of intravenous sugar solutions over a period of time.

By far the most frequent cause of a hypoglycemic reaction occurs in a patient with diabetes mellitus who has taken too much insulin or eaten too little food. Other types of hypoglycemia can be divided into two categories: organic (fasting) hypoglycemia and functional (reactive) hypoglycemia. The more serious of the two, organic hypoglycemia, may be characterized by the central nervous system symptoms described earlier (rather than the adrenaline-release symptoms). It occurs in the early morning before breakfast, after eight to twelve hours without food.

Organic hypoglycemia is much more rare than the functional type and always requires intensive medical investigation to determine the cause. It can usually be diagnosed by detection of a low blood sugar level after an overnight fast. The level of insulin in the blood may also be measured and, if found to be high, an insulin-producing pancreatic tumor is usually the likely cause. Less commonly, other kinds of abdominal tumors may produce insulinlike substances that lower the blood sugar level. In addition, advanced liver disease, congenital liver enzyme defects, chronic adrenal insufficiency, and decreased pituitary function may also cause organic hypoglycemia. Tests that distinguish among these various causes are complicated, but are readily available. These tests are essential for selection of the proper therapy. If organic hypoglycemia is left untreated, or treated improperly, convulsions, coma, and even death can result. Treatment of organic hypoglycemia consists of appropriate therapy for the underlying disease, such as surgical removal of the insulin-secreting pancreatic tumor.

In contrast, an episode of functional hypoglycemia commonly follows a meal—sometimes by as much as three to four hours. Some physicians believe that functional hypoglycemia results from excessive production of insulin by the pancreas in response to an increase in blood sugar. The release of excess insulin abruptly decreases the blood sugar to an abnormally low level, which brings on the hypoglycemic symptoms. In some cases of functional hypoglycemia, however, insulin release has been shown to be normal. Thus, in some people the hypoglycemia may actually be due to an abnormal sensitivity to normal amounts of insulin.

A diagnosis of functional hypoglycemia must be documented by a glucose tolerance test that is *definitely* abnormal. A glucose tolerance test is always taken on an empty stomach. After a small amount of blood is withdrawn from the patient's arm, the patient drinks a measured amount of sugar solution. Blood samples are then taken at hourly intervals for four or five hours and analyzed for sugar. Some physicians also determine insulin levels at each timed interval in the test. The rate of rise and fall of blood sugar is studied, and deviations from normal standards are noted. (A more common form of the glucose tolerance test is the three-hour version, used primarily for the detection of diabetes mellitus, not hypoglycemia.)

During the course of a glucose tolerance test for hypoglycemia the patient must be observed for typical symptoms—the adrenaline-release symptoms mentioned earlier. Most physicians are aware that many normal people—those with no symptoms at all—have what appears at first glance to be a low blood sugar level during the course of the five-hour glucose tolerance test. Many authorities believe this to be an entirely normal phenomenon. In such instances, however, blood sugar rarely falls to less than 45 or 50 milligrams per 100 cubic centimeters of blood. In fact, CU's medical consultants emphasize that only when the blood sugar level falls below 45 milligrams per 100 cubic centimeters can it be said that hypoglycemia does indeed exist.

Relatively few people who complain of nervousness, anxiety, depression and palpitations actually have functional hypoglycemia, according to CU's medical consultants. And those who do experience such symptoms may often have emotional problems. Whether the symptoms are caused by emotional problems, or vice versa, has not yet been resolved. Most endocrinologists believe that many people with one type of functional hypoglycemia are prediabetic and will eventually develop diabetes mellitus, especially if there is a family history of the disease. Another type of functional hypoglycemia may be encountered in individuals who have had stomach operations for peptic ulcer.

Standard treatment for a diagnosed case of functional hypoglycemia generally consists of restricting carbohydrate intake. Low-carbohydrate diets (75–150 grams per day) are prescribed, and the number of daily meals is increased from the usual three to about five or six smaller ones. Carbohydrate restriction as treatment for functional hypoglycemia may seem contradictory, considering that glucose—a carbohydrate—is taken to relieve an acute attack. (Glucose restores blood sugar levels to normal, leading to easing of symptoms.) When used as part of dietary treatment, however, carbohydrate restriction may forestall an excessive release of insulin—and an attack of functional hypoglycemia.

Consumers Union's medical consultants warn, however, that low carbohydrate diets should be prescribed by a physician—and then only after appropriate laboratory tests have documented true functional hypo-glycemia. Unsubstantiated diagnosis or self-treatment could result in unnecessary carbohydrate restriction or inappropriate therapy.

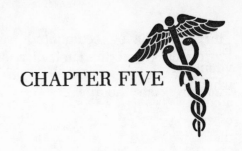

CHAPTER FIVE

The Vitamin E Cure-All

The overpromotion of vitamins is by now a familiar story, but for several decades one vitamin in particular has been singled out by its proponents to be the savior of humanity. Vitamin E is still widely promoted as a preventive, a treatment, or a cure for literally scores of human ailments—ranging from diabetes and heart disease to infertility, ulcers, and warts. It has even been touted as an antidote for air pollution.

Millions of patients, it is alleged, suffer from painful, crippling, life-threatening diseases because their misguided physicians refuse to recommend vitamin E supplements to them. And a generation of children, it is said, is destined in turn to suffer and to die prematurely because they are not receiving daily preventive doses of vitamin E. Such claims as these have appeared in magazine articles as well as in widely circulated paperback books bearing such titles as *Vitamin E for Ailing and Healthy Hearts, Vitamin E: Your Key to a Healthy Heart,* and *Vitamin E: Key to Sexual Satisfaction.*

Are any of these allegations justified? What is vitamin E, and what is it really good for? The beginning of the vitamin E story goes back more than half a century when researchers at the University of California raised a colony of rats on a special diet containing all of the essential nutrients then known. The rats thrived on this diet. They mated normally, and the females became pregnant—but almost all of the fetuses died. When the diet was later supplemented with lettuce or alfalfa, normal offspring were born. Clearly, something essential was missing from the original diet.

In time the missing nutrient was identified as a fat-soluble alcohol, which the discoverers named tocopherol—from the Greek *tokos,* meaning childbirth, and *phero,* to bear or bring forth. Nutritionists called it vitamin E, a term now used interchangeably with alpha-tocopherol, the most biologically potent compound in the tocopherol family. The substance was synthesized in the laboratory in 1938.

Eventually, experimental diets lacking in vitamin E were fed to rats, cattle, sheep, rabbits, dogs, chickens, and other species to find out what would result. The effects varied widely from species to species. In some monkeys, for example, severe lack of vitamin E produced a muscle disease closely resembling a type of human muscular dystrophy. Chickens developed a brain disease, muscular incoordination, and paralysis. Rat livers degenerated, and so did the sperm-producing cells in rat testicles. The hearts of calves were damaged.

This early research indicated that vitamin E is essential for many animal species—and it led to speculation that lack of the vitamin might affect human health.

Vitamin E, accordingly, was tried out on human patients with fertility problems, repeated miscarriages, muscular dystrophy, and other conditions resembling those found in the test animals. The results were for many years uniformly disappointing. No human condition could be identified that benefited from alpha-tocopherol. As a result, vitamin E remained "a vitamin in search of a disease."

In 1953 M.K. Horwitt, M.D., head of the Biochemical Research Laboratory at Elgin State Hospital in Elgin, Illinois, made the first study of what happens when humans are maintained for protracted periods on low-E diets. The project spanned more than eight years —making it one of the longest as well as one of the most thorough studies of human metabolism under controlled conditions. A total of thirty-eight subjects participated in the study.

The outcome of the project can be simply stated: There was no apparent physical or mental impairment caused by the restricted intake of vitamin E. Low-E patients remained in satisfactory health, despite the fact that blood levels of alpha-tocopherol were lowered by 80 percent. The survival time of their red blood cells became somewhat shorter—on the average, about 110 days instead of 123—than that of the two comparison groups (those on a low-E diet who received vitamin E supplements, and those on a standard diet). But the number of cells remained adequate and no patient became anemic. Nevertheless, the shorter survival time was considered sufficient reason for terminating the experiment. In earlier studies monkeys maintained on diets severely deficient in vitamin E had developed anemia, and Horwitt did not want to risk that possibility with the Elgin patients. In short, the study showed that human beings apparently need *some* vitamin E, but that the requirement is a modest one and can be easily satisfied by typical, everyday diets.

Nine patients in the project developed peptic ulcers, which showed up in X-ray examinations although not in patient symptoms. After extensive study, experts in peptic ulcer disease concluded that the ailment was caused by factors other than vitamin E deficiency. Significantly, the incidence of ulcers was no higher among low-E patients than among those who received the same diet plus vitamin E supplements. With standard therapy the ulcers healed without complications. (Despite this experience, vitamin E is still being touted as a treatment for ulcers.)

In 1967 the human need for vitamin E received further confirmation following a study of eleven premature infants who were suffering from hemolytic anemia —early destruction of red blood cells. These babies had been receiving neither cow's milk nor human breast milk but a synthetically concocted commercial milk substitute containing inadequate amounts of vitamin E. On that diet, the anemic babies' blood showed very low levels of alpha-tocopherol. When the babies were given a vitamin E supplement, the hemolytic anemia promptly cleared up. The results were verified in a subsequent controlled trial involving twenty-five premature babies. No longer was vitamin E a vitamin in search of a disease. Those 1967 studies by two Philadelphia physicians, Frank A. Oski and Lewis A. Barness, still provide the best proof that vitamin E is essential in human infant nutrition. As a result of their work, the U.S. Food and Drug Administration began to require that commercial milk substitutes sold as infant foods contain adequate amounts of vitamin E.

But what about adults? Vitamin E enthusiasts claim that millions of Americans, especially those whose intake of polyunsaturated fats is low, don't get enough vitamin E in their diet. The deficit, they insist, should be made up by vitamin E supplements. The fact is, however, as the National Research Council made clear in 1973, that vitamin E is available in adequate quantities in the ordinary diet. According to the NRC, "Dietary vitamin E is supplied in substantial amounts by most vegetable oils as well as by margarine and shortening made from these oils, and significant inputs are made by many vegetables and by whole-grain cereals. Meats, fish, poultry, milk, eggs, legumes, fruits, and nuts also contribute to the dietary supply."

Foods containing polyunsaturated fats are generally high in vitamin E. Margarine made of polyunsurated fats has at least thirteen times more vitamin E than butter. A salmon steak contains ten times the vitamin E of a beefsteak, pound for pound. And most vegetable oils, which are relatively high in polyunsaturated fats, are also adequate sources of vitamin E, despite refining procedures used in processing. In short, when people eat more polyunsaturated fats, their intake of vitamin E is concomitantly increased. Even though there is an increased requirement for vitamin E in a diet high in polyunsaturated fats, that requirement is automatically met. In contrast, when the intake of polyunsaturated fats is low, the need for vitamin E is also low. "The apparent absence of vitamin E deficiency in the general population suggests that the amount of vitamin E in foods is adequate," the NRC pointed out in its 1973 statement.

This conclusion was reinforced by a Food and Drug Administration panel of experts on vitamins and minerals. In a report published in March 1979, the panel included a recommendation against the over-the-counter sale of vitamin E supplements on the grounds that deficiencies of vitamin E are "practically nonexistent." Currently, the Recommended Daily Allowance of vitamin E for adults is 12 to 15 international units, equivalent to approximately 8 to 10 milligrams of natural vitamin E in foods.

Vitamin E proponents sometimes allege that, while ordinary diets may be good enough for ordinary good health, vitamin E supplements may lead to even better health—with greater physical vigor, strength, and endurance. Three researchers in Britain, I. M. Sharman, M.D., M. G. Down, M.D., and R. N. Sen, subjected that possibility to a test. Thirteen boys in a boarding school swimming club were given 400 milligrams of vitamin E daily during a six-week program of intensive physical training. Before and after the six-week period, they were put through a variety of tests—including pull-ups, push-ups, sit-ups, breathholding, running, and swimming endurance. Significant improvement was shown at the end of the six weeks—which might lead some vitamin E enthusiasts to shout "Aha!" But thirteen other boys, matched to the thirteen test subjects in age, weight, and other criteria, had been subjected to the same training program and evaluation. And they had been given an inert medication similar in appearance to the vitamin E capsule taken by the test subjects. The placebo group had also improved. "No significant differences were found between the group given vitamin E and that given placebo tablets," the British researchers reported.

Very low levels of vitamin E have been found in patients with cystic fibrosis, celiac disease, nontropical sprue, chronic pancreatitis, and a few other diseases. These disorders are not caused by lack of vitamin E, however, nor can they be helped by vitamin E. On the contrary, it is the disease that causes the low levels of the vitamin. All of these ailments have one feature in common: an impairment in the small intestine's ability to absorb fat. Consequently, the vitamin E dissolved in that fat is not absorbed either. Even if such patients eat diets with an abundant quantity of vitamin E, very little of it would reach their bloodstream. In these patients, most of the vitamin E consumed, along with most of the fats, is excreted in their stools, a disorder known as steatorrhea. Nor do these patients appear to suffer from their low E levels. Some doctors, however, believe in giving a vitamin E supplement to such patients even though a deficiency state has not been demonstrated.

There is another very special circumstance in which vitamin E may possibly be useful. The vitamin, which functions as an antioxidant, protects fats and other substances from being broken down by oxygen in human beings who, for a variety of reasons, have been exposed to unnaturally high oxygen pressures. The early astronauts, for example, breathed oxygen-enriched air in their space capsules. Hyperbaric chambers containing oxygen under high pressure are sometimes used in treating gas gangrene, carbon monoxide poisoning, and other conditions. The possible value of vitamin E supplements under such circumstances is still speculative, but some doctors believe it merits further investigation.

In 1973 an announcement suggesting that vitamin E protects against harm from air pollutants was hailed with delight by vitamin E fans. The announcement was based on a study published in 1972 in the *Journal of Agricultural and Food Chemistry,* which showed that rats exposed to ozone or nitrogen dioxide were protected from damage when given a vitamin E supplement. What the enthusiasts overlooked was a critical part of the experiment. These were not ordinary rats. They were rats maintained for long periods on artificial diets with such low levels of vitamin E that their stored reserves had been depleted. Under these extreme circumstances, the rats were particularly vulnerable to ozone or nitrogen dioxide toxicity—and raising their vitamin E to *normal* levels protected them. The experiment had nothing whatever to say about the effects of air pollutants on ordinary rats—much less on human beings who eat ordinary, everyday diets. Nor did the authors of the study contend that vitamin E supplements would protect people from air pollution. Yet, results obtained with animals *deprived* of vitamin E were mistakenly applied to human beings. Many claims made for vitamin E rest on precisely the same fallacy.

In addition to the claims made for alpha-tocopherol as a vitamin, the same chemical has for more than a quarter of a century also been touted as a medicine.

Health Quackery

The doses of vitamin E specified in medicinal use commonly range from 300 to 600 milligrams a day or even higher—from thirty to sixty times the Recommended Daily Allowance. It was the news magazine *Time* that first broke the story of vitamin E as a medicine in its issue of June 10, 1946: "Out of Canada last week came news of a startling scientific discovery: a treatment for heart disease (the nation's No. 1 killer) which so far has succeeded against all common forms of the ailment. . . . Large, concentrated doses of vitamin E . . . benefited four types of heart ailment (95 percent of the total): arteriosclerotic, hypertensive, rheumatic, old and new coronary heart disease. The vitamin helps a failing heart. It eliminates anginal pain. It is non-toxic."

The clinical trials that *Time* so enthusiastically recounted were conducted by three physicians—Evan Shute of London, Ontario, a fellow of the American College of Obstetricians and Gynecologists and of the Royal College of Surgeons (Canada); his brother, Wilfrid E. Shute, a specialist in heart disease; and Albert Vogelsang, also of London, Ontario. They based their enthusiasm for vitamin E on their personal experiences with patients. An example reported by Wilfrid E. Shute involved a fifteen-year-old boy who had suffered a second attack of acute rheumatic fever. During his first attack, the boy had been hospitalized for an extended period. This time, however, Shute did not recommend hospitalization. "The only treatment I used for the boy was 200 units of alpha-tocopherol daily," Shute reported. "In three days he was apparently well, and on the sixth day he walked into my office. He was able to return to normal farm activities. . . . This was the first case in all the world in which rheumatic fever had been treated with vitamin E."

This account, of course, aroused worldwide medical interest. It was whetted even further when the Ontario group reported in 1947 on eighty-four Canadian patients treated with vitamin E. According to the group, all of the patients had symptoms of angina pectoris— chest pain usually associated with coronary heart disease—and the majority had improved with vitamin E treatment.

Despite such glowing accounts from Ontario of vitamin E benefits, the vast majority of physicians have rejected vitamin E as a treatment for heart disease. The charge is repeatedly made that the medical profession turned thumbs down on vitamin E without even trying it out. This is simply false. Vitamin E was in fact tried —and found wanting. By 1950 thirteen studies had been published in medical journals, all reporting the worthlessness of vitamin E during clinical trials with patients who suffered from various forms of heart disease. These reports were written by thirty-two researchers, including eminent cardiologists and professors of internal medicine. They involved more than four hundred and fifty patients—as compared with the eighty-four patients on whom Shute, Shute, and Vogelsang based their initial reports.

If any of those thirteen studies had even partially verified the claims made in Canada, further trials of Vitamin E would unquestionably have followed. News of a potential cure for heart disease compels medical attention, and no doctor or scientist would ignore valid evidence in support of vitamin E. "We had indeed intended expanding our studies," a research group at Jewish Hospital in Philadelphia noted in 1948, "but the discouraging results presented in the preliminary report deterred us from carrying these investigations further."

Those sentiments were representative of the medical community at large, as Herbert Eichert, M.D., of Miami, Florida, confirmed during his studies of vitamin E and heart disease in 1948. In an attempt to determine the views of many heart specialists—including those who had not published any findings—Eichert sent questionnaires to medical school department heads throughout the United States. "Most of the clinicians," he reported, "abandoned their trials because of the utter lack of response during the preliminary phases of their investigations." Then, in just one sentence, Eichert summed up all the medical evidence he had gathered on vitamin E's performance: "With the exception of the claims made by Shute and Vogelsang and their group, every published, written, or verbal report which this essayist has been able to obtain indicates that vitamin E has no value in the treatment of heart disease."

Nearly three decades later, researchers evaluating vitamin E for patients with angina pectoris reached essentially the same conclusion. Investigators at the Baltimore U.S. Public Health Service Hospital reported in 1977 that very large daily doses of vitamin E—1,600 international units—produced no measurable improvement in fourteen months of treatment.

In the history of vitamin E research, only a handful

of field trials have complied with the rigorous standards required in compiling scientific data—and most of those trials ended with negative conclusions. The studies by Shute, Shute, and Vogelsang on which claims were made for vitamin E in heart disease were not double-blind experiments—that is, controlled studies in which neither doctor nor patient know which subjects receive the real medicine and which the placebo (until the test is over and all the coded results are in). Indeed, Consumers Union has seen no evidence that the Canadian group even took the essential step of matching patients with controls—let alone the randomization of patients, a requirement of a good study. The findings of the Canadians are essentially the personal impressions of three physicians who had faith in their remedy and who transmitted that faith to their patients. Their claims, in short, are strictly anecdotal and as such have little validity.

Other claims for vitamin E suffer from the same limitations. The Shute brothers, for example, reported that patients with diabetes were able to reduce their daily insulin dose or give up insulin altogether by taking vitamin E. However, it should be pointed out that the Shutes advised those patients to adopt time-honored methods of improving diabetic control, including limitations on their intake of carbohydrates. And the Shutes stressed the importance of complying with such dietary restrictions. As a result, the diabetic patients may well have been able to cut down on their insulin dosage (or, in mild cases, dispense with it altogether). The Shutes' mistake was to attribute their results to vitamin E rather than to their good dietary advice.

Conceivably, the Shute brothers could have discovered that for themselves if they had divided their patients into two groups—giving both the best possible health advice, but supplying vitamin E to one group only. When E. H. Bensley, M.D., and his associates at Montreal General Hospital did that, they found that both groups of diabetics did equally well. The vitamin E was superfluous.

When vitamin E is tested by physicians who are not enthusiasts, the list of failures is long. Clinical trials have failed to show any vitamin E benefits for miscarriages, sterility, menopausal disturbances, muscular dystrophies, cystic fibrosis, blood disorders, leg ulcers, diabetes, and a variety of heart and vascular diseases. The 1973 statement by the National Research Council was also negative about the supposed value of vitamin E supplements for the wide variety of ailments for which vitamin E is promoted.

A few studies suggest that vitamin E might be useful in the treatment of intermittent claudication—a vascular condition in which the blood flow to the lower limbs is reduced and pain, most often in the calves, is experienced during walking. However, the evidence for any such benefit from vitamin E is far from conclusive, in the judgment of Consumers Union's medical consultants who reviewed the studies. The only therapeutic use for vitamin E in human beings established by a well-controlled clinical trial is in the treatment of premature infants who have a rare type of hemolytic anemia caused by a vitamin E deficiency. Beyond that, some doctors prescribe vitamin E as part of an overall therapeutic effort in the treatment of some diseases involving impairment of fat absorption. Vitamin E's value in a high-oxygen environment, which clearly has limited applicability, may possibly be valid but is still not established.

The efficacy of vitamin E in toilet soaps or cosmetics for skin care, despite advertised claims, has not been demonstrated. Its possible advantage in a deodorant was ruled out when the distribution of *Mennen E* was halted by its manufacturer because of an unexpected number of allergic reactions in unhappy users.

Research on vitamin E should continue, CU's medical consultants believe, in order to clarify its role in human metabolism both in healthy people and the sick. Meanwhile, CU's medical consultants discourage, as a waste of money, the use of vitamin E as a dietary supplement or as a medication for common ailments. Apart from the unnecessary expense, such self-medication could lead to postponing proper medical treatment. For now, CU's medical consultants conclude, there is no convincing evidence that human beings need more vitamin E than they obtain in their ordinary diet, or that vitamin E is useful in the treatment of any common disease.

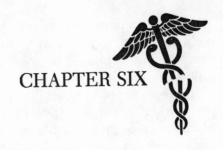

CHAPTER SIX

The Assault on Fluoridation

"There are three kinds of lies," remarked nineteenth-century British statesman Benjamin Disraeli, "Lies, damned lies, and statistics." Probably every type of misrepresentation known to Disraeli, and some he may have overlooked, have been used to attack fluoridation. Misleading information about it appears regularly in a paper called the *National Fluoridation News,* and the entire gamut of hokum has been published in a 176-page issue of the *Cancer Control Journal,* a pro-Laetrile magazine based in Los Angeles. This chapter responds to the lies and false claims that have been made in the attack on fluoridation.

One evening in February 1976, millions of people in Holland were watching television with more than customary attention. News of a bribery scandal in the United States had just reached Europe, along with rumors that Prince Bernhard of Holland was implicated. Those who tuned in were unaware, however, that an unrelated interview later in the newscast would soon affect many of them more directly than the scandal.

The interview involved Dean Burk, Ph.D., an American biochemist formerly with the National Cancer Institute, the federal agency that conducts or sponsors much of the cancer research in the United States. Burk's message was a troubling one. Adding fluoride to drinking water as a dental health measure, he asserted, was causing thousands of cancer deaths annually in the United States. He claimed that statistical studies he had done with another biochemist, John Yiamouyiannis, Ph.D., showed a link between fluoridation and cancer. Burk expressed no reservations about his conclusion. "Fluoridation," he told the television audience, "is a form of public mass murder."

Copies of the Burk-Yiamouyiannis report had been circulated to members of the Dutch Parliament before the television appearance. Soon after, a proposal by the Minister of Health to fluoridate all drinking water supplies in Holland died in Parliament. By September 1976 a Royal Decree ended fluoridation in Rotterdam and in other Dutch cities that had been treating their water for years.

What happened in Holland was not an isolated incident. Despite widespread endorsement of fluoridation by medical, dental, and public health officials, the practice has come under increasing attack both in the United States and abroad as a potential cause of cancer and other diseases. Water fluoridation is the only public health measure that many Americans vote on directly. In 1975, after a publicity campaign linking fluoride to cancer, Los Angeles voters defeated an ordinance to fluoridate the city's water supply. Voters in hundreds of smaller American cities and towns have taken similar action, often out of fear of cancer or other disorders attributed to fluoridation.

How valid are these fears? Is there a genuine scientific controversy surrounding the safety of fluoridation? In 1975 James J. Delaney, who was then a Democratic representative from New York and chairman of the powerful House Rules Committee, responded with an emphatic "yes." A long-time opponent of fluoridation, Delaney urged Congress to halt the practice, pending further investigation of its safety. In the fall of 1977 a subcommittee of the House Committee on Government Operations held hearings on the issue. Burk and Yiamouyiannis testified, as did representatives of the American Dental Association, the National Cancer Institute, and authorities on fluoride research.

What emerged from the testimony, in Consumers Union's opinion, was an unmistakable impression that millions of Americans were being grossly misled about an issue important to both their health and the cost of their dental bills. Yet the House hearings received only scant coverage by the press, except in publications that commonly run antifluoridation stories. Accordingly, in this chapter we will tell you the facts about fluoridation —what it is, how it developed, and what it does.* We will also examine the claims about fluoridation and cancer and consider the people behind those claims. Finally, we'll take a look at other charges frequently lev-

---

*For a discussion of topically applied fluoride in care of the teeth, see the Consumers Union book *The Medicine Show* by the Editors of Consumer Reports Books.

eled at fluoridation, including claims about allergies, birth defects, and heart disease.

Fluorides are compounds containing the element fluorine. In its various forms, fluoride is found in practically all soils, plants, and animals, as well as in human blood, bones, and teeth. It's also present in at least trace amounts in all natural water supplies. The concentration in water varies widely, however. In the United States natural fluoride levels range from a high of about 8 parts per million (ppm) in areas of the Southwest to as little as 0.05 ppm in the Northeast.

Fluoridation is simply an adjustment of the natural fluoride content to about 1 ppm—a level of intake that strengthens tooth enamel and sharply reduces dental decay, especially among those exposed to fluoridated water from early childhood. The nominal 1 ppm level (actually 0.7 to 1.2 ppm, according to local conditions) isn't an arbitrary one. Its selection involved a scientific detective story complete with a twist ending.

The initial clue was uncovered early in the century by two scientists investigating a cosmetic defect. F. S. McKay and G. V. Black were trying to find out what caused a mottling of the tooth enamel, a discoloration variously known as "Colorado brown stain" and "Texas teeth." By 1916 they had narrowed the search to something in domestic water supplies. The next step was to identify the substance and get it out of the water. Not until 1931, however, was the substance identified as fluoride.

Meanwhile, McKay had noticed something else. A practicing dentist, he observed that patients with mottled teeth also had remarkable resistance to tooth decay. The concern of public health officials at the time was still how to get fluoride out of the water. But McKay's observation also spurred further research by the U.S. Public Health Service to learn more about fluoride's effect on teeth.

Over the next ten years, research teams led by H.T. Dean, D.D.S., of the Public Health Service, studied the dental status of 7,257 children in twenty-one cities with various levels of natural fluoride in their water. The results were unequivocal. The more fluoride in the water, the fewer dental cavities the children experienced. When the water contained approximately 1 ppm or more of fluoride, the children developed about 60 percent fewer cavities than did those who drank water with negligible fluoride content. Furthermore, at the 1 ppm level, the unattractive mottling did not occur. It was associated with levels above 2 ppm. Thus, 1 ppm of fluoride became the benchmark level.

Tooth decay was no minor health problem. During the war year of 1942 some 2 million men were examined as potential members of the armed forces. Almost 10 percent of them were rejected because they didn't have twelve sound teeth in proper position, out of a possible thirty-two.

Although the potential dental advantages of fluoridation were obvious, there was then no background of scientific data about possible side effects. There were some practical reassurances, though. People had been ingesting fluoride in food and water since the dawn of the human race. Many Southwesterners had been drinking water containing several times the 1 ppm level of fluoride for a lifetime without any discernible side effects except mottled teeth. Eventually, a few cities decided to take the chance.

Among the pioneers was the New York State Department of Health. Before attempting any widespread introduction of fluoridation, the department proposed a long-term, controlled study of a group of children who would be carefully monitored by physicians. After considering various communities, the department chose the cities of Newburgh and Kingston as ideal candidates for the study. Located some thirty-five miles apart near the Hudson River, both cities had populations of about thirty thousand and were similar in racial, economic, and other demographic characteristics. Each also used reservoirs with water deficient in fluoride.

One city's water supply was to be fluoridated, the other's not. Meanwhile, matched groups of children from the two cities were to be followed from infancy by means of comprehensive pediatric checkups to detect any side effects from fluoride. Special attention was to be given to growth rates, bone development, blood chemistry, the skin, the thyroid gland, vision, and hearing. Each child would also receive meticulous, regular dental examinations.

In 1944 the City Council of Newburgh agreed to participate in the study and approved the fluoridation of its water to 1 ppm. Kingston agreed to serve as the control city and use its fluoride-deficient water without change. A total of 817 children were enrolled in the Newburgh group and 711 in Kingston. Although most entered at the start of the study, several infants were added during each of the first three years to ensure having some children whose mothers were exposed to fluoridated water throughout pregnancy.

The study went on for ten years, and a majority of the children in both groups participated through the final examination. The findings can be summarized briefly: The examinations disclosed no significant medical differences between the two groups that could even remotely be attributed to fluoride. There was one significant dental difference, however. The Newburgh children experienced nearly 60 percent fewer cavities than the Kingston children.

Numerous studies have since confirmed the benefits of fluoridation. "Fewer cavities" means fewer costly multisurface fillings, fewer lost teeth, and, eventually, fewer dentures or partial dentures. The cost of fluoridation to a community, according to a 1977 report in the *New England Journal of Medicine,* is only about ten to forty cents a year per capita. The Public Health Service estimates that this expense amounts to about $1 for every $36 saved in dental bills.

Since the early days of the Newburgh-Kingston project, literally thousands of scientific studies have examined the effectiveness and safety of fluoride. Virtually every doubt or question that has been raised, however scanty the evidence, has been studied in depth by one or more groups of researchers. As a dentist representing the American Dental Association noted in the 1977 House subcommittee hearings, "Fluoridation may well be the most thoroughly studied community health measure of recent history."

In the late 1960s the World Health Organization accomplished the Herculean task of pulling together much of the known information on fluoridation. The objective was to provide an impartial review of the scientific literature on the subject—a vast international aggregation of population studies, experimental research, animal studies, and clinical investigations, including human autopsy studies, clinical trials, and X-ray results.

The report, "Fluorides and Human Health," came out in 1970. It addressed numerous questions raised up to that time about the possible effects of fluoride on different organs and its alleged association with various diseases. The study found no reliable evidence that any ill effects or symptoms resulted from drinking water fluoridated at recommended levels. In a statement issued in 1975, the organization noted: "The only sign of physiological or pathological change in life-long users of optimally fluoridated water supplies . . . is that they suffer less from tooth decay." Since the report's publication, the World Health Organization has uncovered no evidence to alter its judgment.

No amount of study, however, has managed to quiet the criticism of fluoride that has been present from the beginning. Writing in the *Journal of the American Dental Association* in March 1956, Herman E. Hilleboe, M.D., then commissioner of New York State's Department of Health, told of some of the troubles his agency had encountered in the early days of the Newburgh-Kingston project. Soon after the project's approval in 1944, the local health officer in Newburgh began receiving complaints from some of the town's citizens. Some protested that the fluoridated water was discoloring their saucepans. Others complained that it was giving them digestive troubles. One woman complained to her dentist that the "fluoride water" had caused her denture to crack. "These incidents all occurred before fluoride was added to the water supply," Hilleboe noted. After a Newburgh newspaper criticized the town's imaginary ills, the complaints stopped abruptly.

Despite the success of fluoridation in Newburgh, protests against it elsewhere were still vigorous a decade later. The rise of "a vociferous minority," said Hilleboe, had succeeded in delaying, or even reversing, the start-up of fluoridation in several areas. The opposition, he reported, came chiefly from food faddists, cultists, chiropractors, and people who misunderstood what fluoridation was. But the efforts of antifluoridationists have also been aided by the caution of various physicians, dentists, and scientists of good standing who initially questioned the safety of fluoridation. Opposition has also come from other professionals and lay people who view fluoridation primarily as government infringement of individual freedom, an issue beyond the scope of this report.

Various groups have been formed for the sole purpose of fighting fluoridation, but none has had much impact outside of its local community. Generally, the real steam behind the antifluoridation movement has come from well-funded, national, multi-issue organizations that have been able to disseminate large amounts of scare propaganda around the country. One such group is the John Birch Society. Another, up until the early 1970s, was Rodale Press, publisher of *Prevention* magazine and a frequent proponent of unproved nutrition concepts. The most active and effective group today, however, is the National Health Federation, whose roots run deep into the soil of health quackery. Those roots are worth a brief examination.

In the early 1950s, an organization called the Electronic Medical Foundation ran a lucrative diagnosis-by-mail service and also sold electronic treatment devices for "curing" numerous disorders. An estimated three thousand practitioners, mainly chiropractors, would send dried blood specimens from their patients to the foundation. There, the blood spot would be checked by an electronic gadget and a "diagnosis" mailed back by postcard.

This eventually aroused a certain skepticism at the U.S. Food and Drug Administration. Accordingly, the FDA arranged to send a few blood spots of its own. The first, from a man who had lost his right leg, elicited a diagnosis of arthritis in the right foot and ankle. The blood of a dead man brought back a diagnosis of colitis and that of a rooster resulted in a report of sinus infection and bad teeth. The FDA inspectors also investigated the treatment devices. They found that the gadgets simply contained circuits resembling those of an electric doorbell or a small radio transmitter. None could cure anything, reported FDA historian Wallace Janssen.

In 1954 a U.S. District Court ordered the president of the firm, Fred J. Hart, to stop distributing the treatment devices. Shortly thereafter Hart founded the National Health Federation. He continued to distribute the devices, however, and was subsequently prosecuted for criminal contempt and fined $500 in 1962. Between 1957 and 1963, several other NHF officials were convicted of misbranding dietary products with false medical claims and received fines or prison sentences. In 1963 the FDA released a report on the NHF that said in part: "The stated purpose of the federation is to promote 'freedom of choice' in health matters. The record shows that what this frequently means is freedom to promote medical nostrums and devices which violate the law. From its inception, the federation has been a front for promoters of unproved remedies, eccentric theories and quackery."

In a later report on the NHF issued in 1973, the FDA reiterated virtually the same judgment. Throughout its history, the NHF has crusaded against any government interference with unproved remedies or treatments. At the same time, it has also opposed proved public health measures—smallpox vaccination, pasteurization of milk, polio vaccination, and fluoridation of drinking water supplies.

For the most part, the NHF's opposition to public health measures has been a losing cause. Until recent years even fluoridation was slowly gaining acceptance in more communities. About 105 million Americans now have fluoridated water. But in 1974 the NHF decided to mount a new national campaign to "break the back" of fluoridation efforts. It hired John Yiamouyiannis to do the job.

The first big target was Los Angeles, whose City Council had voted in September 1974 to fluoridate the water supply. The NHF's ammunition was a Yiamouyiannis study that purported to link fluoridation to an increase in cancer deaths. The study and a couple of publicity handouts that accompanied it were eventually reviewed by various public health officials, including Thomas Mack, M.D., of Los Angeles, an associate professor of community medicine and an expert in cancer epidemiology. (Epidemiology is a branch of medicine that studies the incidence, causes, and control of a disease in specific populations.) The nature of the Yiamouyiannis study is apparent in an excerpt from Mack's review: "I cannot begin without commenting on the form of the documents you sent me," Mack stated. "Despite the gravity of the question addressed, the form of these sheets is that of a propaganda flyer rather than a serious scientific effort. Specifically, there is no indication that any of the material was ever prepared for submission to a reputable scientific journal. . . . All over the documents one finds . . . conclusions emblazoned essentially in the form of slogans, without cautious interpretation or restrictions. For these reasons, the reader must immediately presume that objectivity has never been considered. . . . At the same time this bias is so pervasive and obvious, the mistaken logic so gross and naive, that the reader assumes the author to be, however competent in his Ph.D. field, totally unaware of the principles of epidemiology."

Most people are unfamiliar with the principles of epidemiology, however, and a Ph.D. degree can sometimes lend credibility even to claptrap. In Los Angeles it evidently did. The scare tactics of the NHF and other antifluoridationists scored a stunning victory over dental health.

Around the beginning of 1975, Yiamouyiannis joined forces with Burk. Like the NHF, Burk is a leading advocate of the worthless cancer drug Laetrile, and he

Health Quackery

shares the NHF's aversion to fluoridation. The collaboration produced a study claiming that twenty-five thousand or more excess cancer deaths occur annually in United States cities that fluoridate their water. The assertion was based on a comparison of death rates for specific cancers in some counties that were fluoridated compared with some that were not. In July 1975 Representative Delaney entered the study into the *Congressional Record* and called for "an immediate suspension of all artificial fluoridation."

The National Cancer Institute reviewed the study and was unimpressed. Unlike a proper epidemiological study, it had failed to take into account widely recognized risk factors known to affect the death rate from specific types of cancers. Using the same data, the NCI reanalyzed the study, taking into account such influences as ethnic composition of the population, geographic location, socioeconomic status, and other significant risk factors. The purported differences in the cancer death rates promptly disappeared.

Undaunted, Burk and Yiamouyiannis bounced back with another study. This time they compared overall cancer death rates for ten large cities with fluoridated water versus ten large cities without fluoridated water. Again, the fluoridated cities came out second best. Over the twenty-year period studied, cancer death rates in the fluoridated cities purportedly increased 10 percent more than in the unfluoridated ones. In December 1975 Delaney entered the second study into the *Congressional Record* and demanded that all fluoridation be stopped.

If anything, the new study was even more amateurish than the July entry. In the judgment of one NCI official at the 1977 House subcommittee hearings, it represented "the worst piece of work that has been done to date on fluoride." Burk and Yiamouyiannis had somehow managed to ignore the most fundamental factors involved in cancer mortality rates—age, sex, and race. Old people die from cancer more often than young people; men have a higher cancer death rate than women; and blacks a higher one than whites. Unless these factors are taken into consideration, the results of a cancer-mortality comparison would be meaningless. When NCI scientists reanalyzed the Burk-Yiamouyiannis data, they found that the difference in the cancer death rate was entirely due to the age and racial makeup of the respective populations. Fluoridation was irrelevant.

Rebuffed by NCI scientists, Burk took the National Health Federation studies to Holland and England. As noted earlier, the Dutch trip was a smashing success. But the British refused to panic. Both the Royal College of Physicians and Oxford University had recently completed studies of fluoridation and cancer. In January 1976 the Royal College of Physicians concluded: "There is no evidence that fluoride increases the incidence or mortality of cancer in any organ." The Oxford study reached a similar conclusion. Moreover, British scientists had learned of the NCI's refutation of the Burk-Yiamouyiannis studies. They also were aware that an independent study conducted for the National Academy of Sciences at the University of Rochester, New York, had confirmed the NCI's findings. "In the normal course of events," reported an Oxford research group, "that would have been the end of the matter. Unfortunately, however, it has not been." What the British scientists hadn't realized was that the facts were only incidental.

The real goal of antifluoridation groups, according to an American Dental Association official, "is to create the illusion of a scientific controversy." The "studies" are merely the ploy. The accuracy of that judgment was proved by what happened next. According to an account in *The Lancet,* a British medical journal, Burk and Yiamouyiannis began publicizing their cancer claims in Britain. Through the assistance of the National Anti-Fluoridation Campaign, their misleading data were circulated to members of Parliament, health authorities, and water boards as evidence that fluoridation was causing many cancer deaths.

Meanwhile, the National Health Federation began claiming in the United States that NCI officials were concealing data, a charge that eventually had an impact in Britain. In Parliament one member accused British health officials of misleading the public about fluoridation and of denying people the truth "because of the Official Secrets Act."

According to testimony at the House subcommittee hearings in 1977, the NCI refused to disclose certain information to the National Health Federation. That refusal, however, was far less sinister than some members of the British Parliament were later led to believe.

The NCI initially gave Burk a copy of the publication "U.S. Cancer Mortality by County: 1950–1969," which he used in preparing the first Burk-Yiamouyiannis report. After the NCI reviewed that report, Yiamouyiannis asked for a copy of the NCI's analyses, which was also dispatched. Then, according to NCI testimony, Yiamouyiannis used that information to attack the NCI's review. Consequently, when he requested a copy of the NCI analyses of his subsequent study, NCI officials denied the request. They pointed out that the basic sources were routine publications of the Bureau of the Census and the National Center for Health Statistics, and they told him, in effect, to do the calculations himself. At the hearings, the NCI's Robert N. Hoover, M.D., said: "The data are generally available to anyone with a public library card."

To check that claim, a Consumers Union staff member visited the local public library. All but two of the volumes needed, both from 1950, were on the shelves of a suburban library within walking distance of our offices. A phone call by a librarian located the two remaining volumes at another nearby branch.

As a result of the charges and the wide publicity the National Health Federation gained in Britain, two British physicians, Richard Doll and Leo Kinlen of the Department of Regius Professor of Medicine at Oxford, decided to undertake still another study. Their reason, they explained, was "to be sure about the truth of the matter, and because we feared that Burk and Yiamouyiannis's abuse of statistics might be detrimental to the future health of British children." At the same time, the Royal College of Physicians requested a formal opinion of the cancer data from the Council of the Royal Statistical Society in Britain.

The resulting studies appeared respectively in 1977 in *The Lancet* and in the *Journal of Applied Statistics.*

Doll and Kinlen reported in *The Lancet* that none of the evidence "provides any reason to suppose that fluoridation is associated with an increase in cancer mortality, let alone causes it." The study conducted for the Royal Statistical Society, which undertook an even more comprehensive statistical analysis than Oxford or the NCI, came to the same conclusion.

Furthermore, additional studies by the NCI in 1976 and subsequent studies by the U.S. Center for Disease Control, the National Heart, Lung, and Blood Institute, and Canada's Health and Welfare ministry each found no evidence linking fluoridation and cancer. In short, independent investigations by eight of the leading medical and scientific organizations in the English-speaking world have unanimously refuted the National Health Federation's cancer claims.

In addition to frightening the public with a baseless claim that fluoridation causes cancer, the opponents of fluoridation have issued many other misleading charges over the years. Fluoridation has been accused of causing ills that range from brittle nails to birth defects. Since such claims are resurrected whenever fluoridation comes up for a vote, we'll discuss the most persistent ones and examine the evidence behind them.

One frequently repeated claim is that fluoride is a poison. Like iron, zinc, and several other minerals, fluorine (in the form of fluoride) is classified by the National Academy of Sciences as an essential trace element in human nutrition. And like many substances essential to life and good health—iron, vitamins A and D, oxygen, and even water itself—fluoride can be toxic in excessive quantities. At high concentrations, fluoride has been used as a poison for insects and rodents. However, at the level in fluoridated water—1 ppm—you'd have to drink at least several hundred gallons at one sitting to get a lethal dose. The water alone would kill you first.

But what about the possibility of slow poisoning—a little bit at a time over long periods? According to the NAS, the daily intake required to produce symptoms of chronic toxicity after years of consumption is 20 to 80 milligrams or more—far in excess of the average intake in the United States. Such heavy doses are associated with water supplies that contain at least 10 ppm of natural fluoride, as in some parts of India. There is absolutely no danger of poisoning from imbibing water fluoridated to prevent dental cavities.

An occasional tactic used in antifluoridation tracts is to print pictures of cattle and other animals harmed by fluoride poisoning. The photographs are authentic, but the impression conveyed is false. Years ago steel mills and clay factories in England and Wales sometimes polluted nearby vegetation with tons of fluoride emissions. Similar incidents have also occurred in this country. Cattle and other animals that grazed on the polluted vegetation would ingest enormous amounts of fluoride and develop bone fractures and lameness. It is pictures of these animals that antifluoridationists use.

A controlled experiment with cattle, however, produced far different results. The cattle were fed various amounts of fluoride in their diet for more than seven years. Even at fluoride levels as high as 27 ppm, the cattle did not experience fractures, lameness, or any adverse effects on soft tissues and milk production. Nor were there any abnormal effects on their offspring through successive generations.

Another common claim is that fluoride causes birth defects. In the late 1950s a French physician named Rapaport reported that Down's syndrome (mongolism) occurred more frequently in some cities with fluoridated water than in some cities with little or no fluoride in their water. Experts who reviewed the study found it seriously flawed, however, especially in its method of locating cases. According to Rapaport's figures, the incidence of Down's syndrome in both the fluoridated and unfluoridated cities was less than half the usual rate—a highly questionable finding in itself. Thus, there was a strong likelihood that Rapaport had failed to uncover the majority of such births in the cities he chose to study.

That conclusion was soon confirmed by a more carefully controlled study in England. Using more exacting methods of case-finding, the British researchers reported that there was no difference in the incidence of Down's syndrome whether the water was high or low in fluoride. Since then, two extensive studies have substantiated the British findings. One surveyed virtually all mongoloid births in Massachusetts from 1950 through 1966. The results, published in the *New England Journal of Medicine* in 1974, showed no link between fluoridation and Down's syndrome. An even larger study published in 1976 covered approximately 1.4 million births in six major United States cities. Researchers at the Center for Disease Control investigated not only Down's syndrome, but also cleft palate, heart abnormalities, clubfoot, and other common birth defects. Again, there was no association between fluoride and any of the defects. In short, the antifluoridationists' claim is based solely on the discredited Rapaport study.

A variation on the birth defects theme is the charge that fluoride is a genetic hazard. Until a few years ago this claim was based on irrelevant or questionable experiments with fruit flies and plants. Then, in 1976, two researchers in Kansas City, Missouri, reported that various levels of fluoride damaged chromosomes in the bone-marrow cells and sperm cells of mice. Although experts who reviewed the experiment noted several inconsistencies in the results, the question it raised was judged important enough to warrant further research.

Accordingly, joint studies were undertaken by the Laboratory of Developmental Biology and Anomalies at the National Institute of Dental Research, the Department of Biochemistry at the University of Minnesota, and the Laboratory of Cellular and Comparative Physiology at the National Institute on Aging. The scientists conducted four separate experiments, including tests on mice receiving acute doses of fluoride and mice raised for several generations on water containing 50 ppm of fluoride. None of the studies produced any evidence that fluoride damages chromosomes, even at levels one hundred times that in fluoridated water supplies.

In Germany, meanwhile, an independent group of researchers reported similar results with human white blood cells, which are especially sensitive to mutagenic agents. Not only did fluoride fail to produce damage, it also exerted an antimutagenic effect by protecting chromosomes against a known mutagen.

Another frequent charge, that people can suffer allergic reactions or "intolerance" to fluoride, gained prominence from anecdotal accounts by George L. Waldbott, M.D., an early opponent of fluoridation who founded the *National Fluoridation News.* Between 1955 and 1965 Waldbott reported numerous instances of patients experiencing nausea, headaches, "spastic colitis," or various other symptoms that he attributed to fluoride ingestion.

In the World Health Organization report described earlier, a review of the Waldbott accounts found no reliable evidence to support his contentions. The cases were judged to represent "a variety of unrelated conditions." The Public Health Service then asked the American Academy of Allergy to evaluate the issue. After a review of the existing clinical reports, the executive committee of the academy concluded unanimously: "There is no evidence of allergy or intolerance to fluorides as used in the fluoridation of community water supplies."

Possibly the most absurd evidence marshaled against fluoridation is material purporting to show that fluoride induces cancer in animals. One series of studies frequently quoted by antifluoridationists was conducted in Texas in the 1950s. The first study involved a strain of mice that ordinarily gets cancer. Supposedly, the mice given fluoridated water developed tumors slightly earlier than similar mice on fluoride-free water. There were a few minor hitches in the experiment, however. All of the mice were also fed a dog chow that, unknown to the investigator, contained 42 ppm of fluoride—or ten to one hundred times the amount any of the mice got in their water, thus making any comparison between the two groups invalid. A further botching occurred when the investigator miscalculated the amounts of fluoride in the water. Two scientists from the National Institutes of Health reviewed the study in 1951 and dismissed it. Other experiments by the same Texas investigator and a co-worker have long been discredited by subsequent research. Nevertheless, opponents of fluoridation still cite the Texas experiments as significant evidence that fluoride is carcinogenic.

Another study that has received star billing in antifluoridation tracts is an experiment conducted with fruit flies in 1963. This time, legitimate findings have been substantially distorted. In the 1963 study, two strains of fruit flies exposed to 20 to 50 ppm of fluoride in their food experienced an increased incidence of melanotic tumors. Opponents of fluoridation interpret that to mean that fluoride can cause cancer. Not so, say scientists at the National Cancer Institute. While human beings may be physiological cousins to the mouse and other mammals, kinship to the fruit fly is somewhat more distant.

Specifically, a melanotic tumor in a fruit fly is not the same as a cancerous tumor in a human or mammal. It is more akin to scar tissue, and, unlike a cancerous tumor, it's not malignant or harmful. It can be induced by a wide range of substances, including some vitamins and even lysine and tryptophan, two amino acids essential for human growth and health. Fruit flies can also get malignant tumors, but there's no evidence that fluoride has ever caused any. Indeed, fluoride has never proved to be carcinogenic in tests on a variety of animals, including mice, rats, hamsters, guinea pigs, rabbits, dogs, and sheep.

In Wisconsin opponents of fluoridation have often charged that it increases the number of deaths from heart disease. They base their claim on statistics that show a rise in heart deaths in the Wisconsin town of Antigo since the introduction of fluoridation there. The National Heart and Lung Institute has called the data a "misrepresentation of statistics." According to one scientist, "The well-known fact that deaths from heart disease become more frequent as people grow older was overlooked." Since fluoridation was introduced in Antigo in 1949, the percentage of elderly people there has doubled. Between 1950 and 1970, for example, the segment of the population seventy-five years old and older increased 106 percent. When this factor is taken into account, the alleged effect of fluoride on heart deaths vanishes.

According to a 1972 study by the National Heart and Lung Institute, comparisons of data from fluoridated and unfluoridated communities reveal no difference in the rate of heart deaths. Furthermore, reported the institute, evidence from autopsy studies, from examinations of people exposed to acute doses of fluoride in industrial accidents, and from medical data on people who have drunk water naturally high in fluoride for a lifetime "all consistently indicate no adverse effect on cardiovascular health." The 1972 conclusions have since been confirmed by large-scale studies conducted by the Center for Disease Control and the National Heart, Lung, and Blood Institute.

Of all the numerous ills that have been attributed to fluoridation—from cancer in human beings to constipation in dogs—no claim has ever been shown to be valid. In fact, the only known hazard of fluoridated water has nothing to do with drinking it. Patients undergoing dialysis for kidney disease can be exposed to about fifty to one hundred times the amount of fluid consumed by the average person. Accordingly, the National Institute of Arthritis and Metabolic Disease recommends that fluoride—as well as calcium, magnesium, and copper— be removed from tap water before it is used in an artificial kidney machine. Aside from that precaution, there is no genuine reason to worry about fluoridation.

In 1960, however, the residents of Antigo, Wisconsin, didn't realize that scare stories being circulated by local opponents of fluoridation were false. Antigo voted to discontinue its eleven-year practice of fluoridating the water supply. The decision eventually led to a study by public health officials, who wanted to learn what effects the end of fluoridation would have on the dental health of Antigo youngsters.

During 1960 dental personnel from the Wisconsin Division of Health examined nearly all children in the kindergarten, second, fourth, and sixth grades of Antigo's schools. The examiners recorded the number of decayed, missing, and filled teeth for each child. Four years later, they repeated the examination among children in all of the same grades except the sixth. The kindergarteners in 1964 had a rate of

119

dental problems 92 percent higher than their coun-
terparts four years earlier. Among second-graders,
the decay rate in permanent teeth was up 183 percent. Among fourth-graders, it was up 41 percent.
Later, an examination of sixth-graders showed a 91
percent increase in decay rates. In 1965 Antigo
voted to reinstate fluoridation.

Despite persisting claims about heart deaths by
local antifluoridationists, today the people of Antigo
still drink fluoridated water. Meanwhile, about 100
million Americans do not, largely because of the
fears raised by opponents of fluoridation. The simple
truth is that there's no "scientific controversy" over
the safety of fluoridation. The practice is safe, eco-
nomical, and beneficial. The survival of this fake controversy represents, in Consumers Union's opinion,
one of the major triumphs of quackery over science
in our generation.

Editors' Note: A few months after CU published its
most recent report about fluoridation (CONSUMER RE-
PORTS, July and August 1978), CU began receiving telephone inquiries from newspaper reporters and public
officials in various parts of the country. In each instance,
the caller was from an area or a city in which fluoridation was an issue in a public hearing or in an upcoming
vote. Invariably, the question was the same: Was it true
that CU was being sued for libel because of our fluoridation report?

It was true. John Yiamouyiannis of the National
Health Federation had instituted an $8 million libel suit

against CU. He charged that he had been defamed by CU's report, which had criticized as baseless and misleading his claims that fluoridation causes cancer.

According to the people who called us, the existence of the libel action against CU was mentioned by opponents of fluoridation whenever CU's report was quoted or introduced at public hearings and local debates on the issue. The lawsuit was apparently being used to some extent as a public relations ploy: Antifluoridationists were saying that CU was being sued, thereby implying that our report was untruthful or biased.

Any publicity value was short-lived, however. In May 1979 Judge Richard Owen of the United States District Court for the Southern District dismissed the suit against CU. In his decision, Judge Owen stated: "... the suggestion is strong that the plaintiff's object in bringing this action is to use this court to discourage the publication of opposing views."

Yiamouyiannis had contended that CU, in its two-part report, had been guilty of "actual malice," a legal term meaning that the material had been published either with knowledge that it was false or with reckless disregard for whether it was false or not. In opposition, CU filed a motion for summary judgment, seeking dismissal of the complaint as meritless.

In support of that motion, CU submitted several affidavits, including extensive documentation of the facts in the report and a description of CU's research and review procedures for the report.

In granting summary judgment in favor of CU and against Yiamouyiannis, Judge Owen said: "There is overwhelming evidence in defendant's affidavits, unrebutted by plaintiff, that the articles were prepared in a conscientious and professional manner after a thorough review of reputable sources and standard reference works on medicine and science. No serious question is raised that either the author or the editors who reviewed and approved the articles for publication had the slightest doubt as to their truth and accuracy."

Yiamouyiannis appealed the decision, and the case was then argued before the United States Court of Appeals for the Second Circuit. In March 1980, the court issued a unanimous opinion upholding Judge Owen's decision. In its opinion, the Court of Appeals reached a conclusion similar to that of Judge Owen's regarding the quality of investigation and preparation involved in CU's report:

"It is clear that [Consumers Union] . . . made a thorough investigation of the facts. Scientific writings and authorities in the field were consulted; authoritative scientific bodies speaking for substantial segments of the medical and scientific community were investigated. The unquestioned methodology of the preparation of the article exemplifies the very highest order of responsible journalism: the entire article was checked and rechecked across a spectrum of knowledge and, where necessary, changes were made in the interests of accuracy."

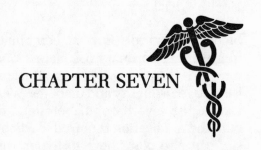

CHAPTER SEVEN

Overweight: Diets, Drugs, and Devices

Humorist Art Buchwald once suggested that the word "diet" comes from the verb "to die." And anyone whose commitment to weight loss has fallen victim to hunger pangs, headaches, fatigue, dizziness, or just plain boredom might well agree. Most overweight people have discovered that losing weight—and maintaining weight loss—is no easy matter. The frequent failure of standard low-calorie diets to overcome obesity in any permanent way has spawned a profusion of fad diets, appetite-suppressing drugs, and reducing gadgets. Unfortunately, most of these measures slenderize only one's bank account. And some may introduce health complications of their own.

Meanwhile, the widespread prevalence of obesity in the United States tends to affect the incidence or severity of several diseases that Americans commonly experience. Obesity itself is not a primary risk factor in coronary heart disease, as are hypertension (high blood pressure), cigarette smoking, and elevated levels of blood cholesterol. But, in combination with one or more of these primary risk factors, obesity substantially increases the chance of heart attack. A relationship exists between obesity and diabetes: Weight loss can often reduce the severity of diabetes and decrease or eliminate the medication required for diabetic control. Obesity can also contribute to hypertension, and at least one form of pulmonary disease is known to be caused by excessive overweight. Obesity has been associated with varicose veins, back troubles, gallbladder stones, and arthritis of the hips and knees.

For many obese people, these common medical complications provide compelling reasons for weight reduction. Beyond such medical implications, moreover, the physical discomfort or psychological burden of massive overweight can also fan the desire to lose weight. Even among those who are only moderately overweight, the trim figure or lean physique constantly promoted in advertising as the contemporary ideal may be reason enough for people to want to shed ten or fifteen extra pounds. For millions of Americans, though, shedding pounds—and keeping them off—tends to be far more difficult than gaining pounds and keeping them on.

It was only in the past decade or two that medical researchers began to provide some clues to the reasons why so many people tend to be overweight. In the mid-1960s pioneering efforts by Jules Hirsch, M.D., and his colleagues at the Rockefeller Institute for Medical Research (now Rockefeller University) in New York City led to the first breakthrough in understanding the nature of obesity. Hirsch and his co-workers were able to show that the fat patient not only had extra-large fat cells, but also an increased number of these cells. As patients lost weight on a low-calorie diet, the *size* of each fat cell decreased, but the *number* of fat cells remained the same. And when patients returned to previous weight levels, each fat cell regained its previous size.

The researchers established that the number of fat cells in each individual remains constant from about puberty onward. Using experimental animals, the study group determined the number of fat cells during the first few weeks after birth. That number was destined to remain fairly constant for the life of the animal. An animal that was relatively deprived of nourishment at that critical time of life tended to become a thinner mature animal than its well-fed littermate. It is believed likely that these observations in animals apply to human beings as well.

The plump child, whose rounded cheeks traditionally symbolized good health, may be the precursor of the obese adult. Many pediatricians, alert to current thinking about origins of obesity, make a serious attempt to limit the caloric intake of young patients. Decreasing the calories consumed in childhood may prevent a disproportionate increase in the number of fat cells and thus possibly spare the child the plight of trying to cope with the problem of obesity in later years.

Environmental influences play an important part in the problem. Widespread advertising of calorie-rich (and often nutrition-poor) foods whet the appetite. The business lunch, the testimonial dinner, the television snack, and the family get-together that focuses on eat-ing—all can contribute to obesity.

Genetic as well as environmental factors may also be involved in the evolution of the obese adult. The child with two obese parents has a greater chance of becom-ing obese than the youngster with only one overweight parent. Least likely to suffer from obesity is the child of two thin parents.

To some extent, economic factors are also involved. Studies have shown that among females it is the woman of means who tends to be thinner than her less affluent sister. Nor can ethnic or national custom be ruled out as a contributor to obesity. Certain people, notably those of Italian and Jewish origin, tend to be more obese than those of Anglo-Saxon background.

Research into the origin and nature of obesity is still in the beginning stages. The causes of obesity are so subtle that they still defy full description. Two thousand calories a day may put weight on one individual and not on another, even though the two have the same body build and seem to engage in similar activities. So no printed chart can be relied on to indicate the optimum number of calories a day. It is not difficult, however, to determine one's proper food intake. Under ordinary circumstances, an adult whose weight is about right should eat the amount that permits maintaining that weight with little or no gain or loss. If weight begins to rise or is too high to begin with, it is time to cut down on total calorie intake. The whole problem of weight control is as simple—or as difficult—as that.

Overeating has many causes. The overwhelming ma-jority of Americans now sit at work or at school, but national food habits stem largely from days when hard physical labor was common. A heavily laden table, in those days a necessity, is now about as useful as a buggy whip. Glandular disorders, often blamed for gross overweight, are actually quite rare. Hypothyroidism, one of the more common endocrine diseases, is the true cause of obesity in only a tiny fraction of the overweight population.

Stomach contractions leading to hunger sensations are unconditioned, primitive reflexes related to the preservation of life. The satisfaction of hunger does not lead to overeating—or to overweight. Appetite, however, is a complex, conditioned drive having both physiological and psychological components. Appetite is based on learning, on the memory of disappearance of hunger sensations and of their replacement by the pleasurable sensations of satiety, well-being, and relaxation. Appetite is also related to the agreeable taste, smell, and appearance of food. It is appetite that induces people who have satisfied their hunger with meat, bread, and vegetables to eat an appealing dessert. And in order to bring down food intake, it is appetite rather than hunger that must be curbed.

Some people who are very concerned about weight reduction might be better off accepting their present weight level. It is certainly best to keep the weight at or slightly below the ideal for one's size, age, sex, and body build, but Consumers Union's medical consultants believe that those who are no more than about 15 percent overweight are better off doing nothing than repeatedly going on and off reducing diets.

It is true that some reducing aids can bring about

temporary reduction in weight, probably in large part because their use helps to put the overweight individual in the proper frame of mind to cut down on intake of food. Unfortunately, it is long-term, not short-term, weight reduction that counts, and the key to that is lowered calorie intake and regular exercise over a period of years. Even such controlled treatment fails much of the time because obesity so often stems from emotional and personality problems associated with eating patterns acquired over a lifetime—problems that are not easily changed. It is extremely rare that a shortcut approach to weight reduction brings about permanent weight control.

Fad Diets

Despite the realities, the promise of a "new" or "effortless" way to lose weight quickly attracts attention. A staple fare of the magazine world is the monthly article touting the latest wonder diet. Readers disillusioned with the grapefruit diet, weary of bouncing from the vegetarian diet to the Stone Age meat diet, or from the gourmet's diet to the brown-bag diet can still try their luck with the thirty-day countdown diet, the nine-day wonder diet, or the twenty-four-hour easy diet. When those fail, dieters can eat themselves slim—and fat again—the French way, seek solace in the pray-your-weight-away diet, or turn to a wide array of books promoting equally foolproof schemes for easy weight loss.

"An endless succession of dietary regimens appears in the media, each purporting to be the ultimate solution," observed George V. Mann, M.D., of Vanderbilt University in *The New England Journal of Medicine.*

"These permutations of fuel mixtures range from the impossible to the ridiculous. If they have any common feature it is that they make elaborate promises of success, they understate the rigors of adherence, and they try to place the decision for dietary restriction in the hands of the dieter. . . . The other common feature of reducing regimens is their commercialism—someone stands to make money from their promotion."

As Mann suggested, the benefits of such regimens seem to accrue primarily to the authors, publishers, and booksellers. Moreover, the readers can sometimes be deprived of more than their money, since some of the fad diets espoused in these books may endanger a person's health.

A typical diet book—and a commercial success in 1973—was *Dr. Atkins' Diet Revolution,* which prescribed a low-carbohydrate regimen. The Medical Society of the County of New York called the diet "unscientific" and "potentially dangerous." The aim of the diet was to produce ketosis, a condition in which fats are burned incompletely, resulting in the appearance of so-called ketone bodies in the blood and subsequently in the urine. Most diets promoting ketosis are likely to produce fatigue, dehydration, and, in some instances, nausea and vomiting. They can also provoke attacks of gout and, in some people, irregular heart beats. Some dieters have noted striking elevations in cholesterol levels. Pregnant women, especially, are warned to avoid this diet. In fact, CU's medical consultants strongly discourage any strenuous dieting, especially low-carbohydrate regimens, during pregnancy. The ketosis that may result has been linked to subsequent mental retardation in children born to mothers on such diets.

"Revolution" was hardly an accurate descriptive title for Atkins's diet. The familiar *Drinking Man's Diet*, published in 1964, was also based on a low-carbohydrate scheme—with added attractions, of course. And before that, another low-carbohydrate diet was advocated by Herman Taller in *Calories Don't Count*, published in 1961. It sold well over a million copies with many of the copies no doubt bought by those who interpreted the title to mean that dieters could eat all the food they wanted. Those buyers were disappointed. Taller advocated a high-fat, low-carbohydrate diet, excluding not only sweets and starches but also most fruits and vegetables. His only evidence of the diet's success was his own experience and the anecdotal experiences of some patients.

Over the years, many "new and revolutionary" diets have been promoted to the unwary—the milk diet, the milk and banana diet, the milk and corn-oil drink, the high-fat diet, the high-protein diet, and other variations and formulations variously called the Hollywood diet, the Du Pont diet, the Rockefeller diet, the *Good Housekeeping* or *McCall's* diet, and recently the Scarsdale diet. In most cases, any weight loss from such diets has been about as fleeting as their fame.

To date, however, none has had such somber results as the liquid protein diet, which first gained popularity in the summer of 1976 with the publication of *The Last Chance Diet* by Robert Linn, a Pennsylvania osteopath. The regimen was touted as the diet of choice "when everything else fails." Linn claimed that the diet "can and should be your last diet. Period." For some people, unfortunately, those words were destined to become a tragic prophecy. The U.S. Food and Drug Administration and the Center for Disease Control have received reports of sixty deaths associated with the liquid protein regimen.

What happened—and why it happened—is important to anyone who wants to lose weight safely. Some of the latest diet aids being promoted claim to be wholly different from the liquid protein products that were hawked earlier, and physically they are. But their marketing thrust—that a specific *product* is the key to a successful diet—is similar to the sales pitch of virtually all diet-aid concoctions, including liquid protein. Accordingly, what happened in the case of the "Last Chance" diet offers insight into how the marketplace often misleads the dieter.

The Last Chance Diet

The regimen popularized by *The Last Chance Diet* consisted only of a few ounces of liquid protein daily, plus vitamin and mineral supplements and noncaloric drinks. It had an element singularly lacking in all other fad diets: a background of serious clinical research and demonstrated results. Under somewhat similar programs conducted at two separate hospitals, severely obese patients had been able to lose massive amounts of weight. The hospital-based programs used an approach known as the "protein-sparing modified fast." Thus, unlike most authors of fad diets, Linn was popularizing a concept that had some basis in fact. However, the modified fast was anything but a diet for the general public. The medical researchers who investigated and developed the approach—principally at Cleveland's Mount Sinai Hospital and the New England Deaconess Hospital in Boston—were primarily engaged in treating patients whose extreme obesity contributed to serious or even life-threatening illness. Typical patients included people with unstable diabetes, hypertension, heart disease, and those whose obesity endangered their chances for successful surgery.

Moreover, none of the patients was merely trying to reduce from a size 16 to a size 12. At the Cleveland hospital, for example, an initial study involving seventy-five patients was limited to persons who were at least 50 percent above their ideal weight. On entering the program, the subjects ranged in weight from 176 to 540 pounds, and the average patient was 96 percent overweight. Virtually all of them had been referred to the program after repeated failure to lose weight by conventional methods.

The reason for limiting admission to the massively obese was simple. Fasting for more than a few days can be dangerous. After a day or two on a total fast, the body begins to burn not only its fat stores but protein tissue as well. And that protein comes from lean body mass—muscles and major organs such as the heart and kidneys. The fast, when prolonged, may also lead to anemia, impairment of liver function, kidney stones, mineral imbalances, and other possible side effects.

The theory behind the modified fast is to supply just enough protein or other nourishment to prevent the body from cannibalizing its own lean tissue. But even so, such a fast represents a major departure from the

body's normal sources of energy, which are mainly carbohydrates.

Accordingly, the modified fast was viewed by its
originators as a relatively severe form of treatment for
obesity, but one that was justified in cases where the
potential benefits outweighed the risks. To minimize
the risks, the medical researchers at the Mount Sinai
and New England Deaconess hospitals took extensive
precautions. Initially, patients were hospitalized for a
week or more for comprehensive clinical evaluation,
including complete history and physical examination,
blood chemistry, urinalysis, and other diagnostic tests.
They were then closely monitored as outpatients during the weight-loss program and thereafter.

Their diets, which amounted to only several hundred
calories daily, were carefully calculated according to
body weight. Generally, they included lean beef, milk
protein, egg white, or other high-quality protein. In
some regimens, protein was used exclusively; in others,
it was combined with carbohydrates, such as glucose or
ordinary sugar. In all instances, though, supplements of
vitamins and minerals, including potassium and calcium, were part of the daily fare.

The program, in short, wasn't something that could
be bottled or canned and sold over the counter. As
practiced at Mount Sinai and New England Deaconess,
it involved close medical supervision of patients by
clinicians experienced in obesity treatment. And it emphasized not only diet, but an overall approach that
included appropriate exercise, instruction in nutrition,
and counseling in behavior modification.

Since 1971, when clinical trials of the modified fast

began, several studies have reported impressive results. One report that appeared in *The Journal of the American Medical Association* in November 1977, for instance, described the experience of 519 patients treated in the Mount Sinai program. Of those patients, 78 percent lost a minimum of forty pounds during the course of the fast. The average patient spent about thirty weeks on the fast and lost approximately three pounds a week.

Such results have encouraged some clinicians to view the fast as a promising method for treating severe obesity, which is usually resistant to conventional weight-loss techniques. Some researchers also believe that properly supervised programs may eventually be applicable for moderately obese patients as well. But a number of questions remain. One is whether a very low calorie diet based on protein is really any better than a mixed diet that's equally low in calories. Some reports, for example, characterize the protein diet as being helpful in appetite suppression. But, as yet, there's no scientific evidence that either diet is superior to the other.

A more crucial question is whether such programs will be successful in the long run. Essentially, can they prepare an obese patient for a lifetime of caloric restriction? Addressing that point in an editorial in *JAMA*, Victor Vertes, M.D., an originator of the Mount Sinai program, summed up the problem: "Unfortunately, as with other weight-reduction techniques, the value of supplemented fasting is limited unless the patient is prepared to modify his life-style and eating habits for maintenance of weight loss. Therefore, we can only endorse supplemented fasting as phase 1 of a two-phase program," said Vertes. "The second and more important phase is maintenance of weight reduction, which requires a long-term commitment from both patient and physician."

Finally, how safe are such programs? Both Vertes and George L. Blackburn, M.D., of the New England Deaconess program, believe that, for selected patients under the right conditions, modified fasting is safe. Those conditions, according to Blackburn, include a properly supervised, comprehensive program conducted by physicians who are knowledgeable in the method.

As yet, the people who have been treated under such conditions number only a few thousand. The potential total of obese candidates, however, numbers well into the millions. Accordingly, Consumers Union's medical consultants believe it is still too early to pronounce a verdict on the safety of the fast in a large population. For the present, say CU's consultants, the method should probably be limited to further clinical trials among the severely obese.

Constraints that govern the medical scientist, however, are often far removed from the ring of the cash register. In contrast to some of the diet-aid entrepreneurs who came soon after, Robert Linn did emphasize in *The Last Chance Diet* the major cautions and components of the modified fast. Readers learned of the need for medical supervision, the importance of a comprehensive approach to weight control, and the crucial role of developing sensible eating habits after completing the diet. But, in the leap from the medical journals to the pages of the book, a curious thing happened: A new elixir was born. It was called *Prolinn* (presumably from *pro*tein and *Linn*) and was eventually to sell for $10 to $16 a quart. No such product was used in the fasting programs at Mount Sinai or New England Deaconess. But suddenly it became an indispensable part of the "Last Chance" diet. "This formula is necessary for the program to work properly," Linn claimed in his book.

Thus was born the "liquid protein" diet, an identical twin of the "Last Chance" diet. But there was little family resemblance to the diets used by Vertes and Blackburn in their modified-fast programs. Blackburn, it's true, had used a formula that contained crystalline amino acids (the chief components of proteins) for intravenous feeding of some surgical patients. But, he said, it was "drastically different" from the stuff used in *Prolinn* or any of the subsequent liquid-protein products. The amino acids in the intravenous solution were produced and compounded in an entirely different way and were of much higher quality, Blackburn told CU. Moreover, the solution included twenty-two other nutrients, such as vitamins and minerals. The liquid proteins generally do not. And some of the amino acids in the liquid proteins "have no value to the body," Blackburn added. "They're merely excreted."

What, then, is liquid protein? Essentially, it's a byproduct of slaughterhouse offal. According to the Food and Drug Administration, it is made by processing the fibrous collagen tissue from animal hides, tendons, and bones—the same substances that were once commonly used for making furniture glue. The process produces a syrupy gelatin of negligible nutritional value. To make it usable by the body, it is then fortified with tryptophan, one of the essential amino acids missing from gelatin. Preservatives are also added, along with flavorings to disguise the taste.

Fueled by sales of *The Last Chance Diet* in 1976, the liquid protein concept caught on quickly. *Prolinn* was soon followed by a host of other brands very similar in composition. For diet-aid entrepreneurs, the liquid protein idea arrived like rain in a drought. Despite the booming market for so-called health and beauty aids— which include drugs, cosmetics, and toiletries—diet-aid products had not sold well. Between 1967 and 1976, sales of health and beauty aids soared 94 percent to a total of $21.5 billion. During the same period, diet-aid sales dropped by some $16 million to their lowest dollar volume in a decade.

Accordingly, the arrival of a new elixir presented an opportunity not to be missed. Dozens of brands of liquid protein quickly appeared, often heavily promoted. But the concept of the modified fast—and the caution with which it should be used—tended to be ignored in the ads we saw. The product would "stop hunger signals" and "change your heavy body chemistry to a slim body chemistry," said a typical mail-order ad. It was the *product* that was emphasized.

By the end of 1977, the liquid protein bandwagon had come to a screeching halt. The reports of deaths among people on the diet had sent sales plummeting, and the FDA took action to ban or regulate the marketing of protein diet aids.

Meanwhile, the makers of widely promoted protein

powders (which are marketed as replacements for one or two daily meals) began taking action of their own. In an attempt to separate their product from liquid protein in the public mind, they ran full-page newspaper ads making a strong promotional bid to replace the scare-tainted liquids.

The powders that were stocked at most stores in CU's area generally turned out to be the brands that were advertised nationally. CU purchased four of them in 1977 for label evaluation—*NaturSlim, P-86 Instant Protein Powder, Slim-Fast,* and *Ultrathin*—and we compared their price, protein content, and other features. We also checked them against some common foods high in protein. All four contained milk protein, and all except *Slim-Fast* contained soy protein as well. All were fortified with various vitamins and minerals. Their outstanding feature, however, was their price. In terms of the amount of protein they supplied, all were more expensive than either sirloin steak or standing ribs of beef. Indeed, the cheapest among them *(P-86)* cost about 40 percent more than sirloin on the basis of protein content. On the same basis, *NaturSlim* was twice the price of sirloin and *Slim-Fast* was nearly four times as much.

When the products were compared with eggs or less expensive meats, such as beef liver or chicken, the disparity was even wider. For the same amount of protein, *Slim-Fast* cost eleven times the price of beef liver. *Slim-Fast,* a "milk-shake" mix, was intended to be used with skim milk. But it was the skim milk that supplied about two-thirds of the protein. The three other powders could be used with fruit juices, milk, and similar beverages. No matter how the powders were to be used, though, they were an exceptionally expensive way to obtain protein.

Nor did they save many calories compared with ordinary food. For example, getting the same amount of protein from *Ultrathin* as that supplied by a 6½-ounce can of tuna in water required 7½ servings (fifteen rounded teaspoons), or 225 calories worth of powder. That saved a whopping 15 calories over the can of tuna —at more than double the price. Mixed with 8 ounces of skim milk, *Slim-Fast* provided about 14 grams of protein—the same amount as in a half-cup of cottage cheese. But that milk shake amounted to about 205 calories, 85 more than the cottage cheese.

Virtually every authority on obesity stresses the need to modify old eating habits to maintain any successful weight loss. Using a protein powder—or any protein supplement—to replace one or two daily meals during a diet is unlikely to prepare people for more sensible eating habits when they reach their intended weight. Consequently, the supplement approach may only serve to keep dieters on what's called the "yo-yo" cycle of weight control.

Other Diet Products

In addition to protein supplements, a variety of other dietary products have been promoted over the years for do-it-yourself reducing. Among the most common types have been formula diets, diet candies, and bulk producers.

For several years, formula diets such as *Metrecal* and *Slender* have been standard items on supermarket shelves. Eventually, the original powders and liquids grew into product lines that include cookies, wafers, and soups. Using such ingredients as skim milk, sugar, vegetable oil, and an assortment of vitamins and minerals, the formula products attempt to duplicate a well-balanced diet yielding about 900 calories daily.

Basically, the formula diets offer the advantages of simplicity and convenience of preparation. However, virtually anyone restricting intake to 900 calories daily could expect to lose weight. A major disadvantage, though, is the monotony of the menu. Few people can tolerate living exclusively on a formula diet for more than a few weeks. Although promoters claim that the formulas are balanced, if the regimen is followed conscientiously for a prolonged period, there is a risk that the dieter may become deficient in one or more essential nutrients supplied by ordinary foods. What's more, chronic diarrhea can also be a problem.

No one should go on any diet as restricted as 900 calories without first checking with a physician. With medical approval, there is no harm is starting a weight-reduction program based on a formula diet, provided the limitations described above are borne in mind. Overall, CU's medical consultants believe that in the long run the use of carefully selected standard foods, combined with regular exercise, is superior to any regimen based on a formula diet product.

While a formula diet offers some limited advantage to those seeking convenience, before-meal candies appear to provide no benefit whatsoever to dieters. These special candy caramels, which are sold under a number of different trade names (*Ayds* is one of the best-known brands), are supposed to suppress appetite and thereby help to control weight. The theory behind these products is that, if the level of sugar in the blood is raised just before meals, the appetite will diminish and the dieter will have no trouble at all giving up rich sauces and gravies, or passing up desserts.

One leading brand of diet candy, when CU checked in 1979, yielded about 25 calories per caramel. The directions advised that two candies be taken before meals—the equivalent in calories to about three teaspoonfuls of sugar, an amount that actually has little effect on the blood sugar level. There is no evidence that before-meal candies suppress appetite.

Remember that when any reducing aid (candy or other) is promoted for use with a stated diet-and-exercise plan, any weight reduction achieved will more than likely be the result of the diet and exercise rather than of the reducing product.

Reducing confections often contain vitamin and mineral supplements. Yet a moderate weight-reducing diet as low as 1,200 calories per day can be well balanced with respect to proteins, vitamins, and minerals; it can include green and yellow vegetables, skim milk or cottage cheese, eggs, lean meat, fish, fowl, fruits, bread, and cereals. Excluding foods excessivily high in calories does not in some mysterious way create a need for extra vitamins and minerals.

Another common diet aid is the bulk producer. Bulk-producing products expand when they absorb water. Taken about ten to thirty minutes before meals, they are supposed to swell up in the stomach and diminish hunger contractions. Typical of the bulk producers is the vegetable product known as methylcellulose. Originally promoted for treatment of constipation, it is now sold to reduce appetite, sometimes in combination with certain central nervous system stimulants (see below). Dieters should bear in mind that these products, if taken in larger than recommended doses, can have a laxative effect.

Methylcellulose and similar bulk producers tend to pass fairly rapidly into the small intestine, especially when taken on an empty stomach. Even while they are in the stomach, there is no clear evidence that their presence really affects the stomach's hunger contractions. And even if hunger contractions were diminished, this would have no bearing on the exaggerated appetite that is the major cause of overeating in obesity.

Appetite-Suppressing Drugs

Until 1971 the most important group of appetite-suppressing agents, from the standpoint of sales, were sympathomimetic amines, drugs that stimulate the central nervous system. In 1971 slightly more than 26 million prescriptions (initial and refills) were filled for these drugs, which have the property of affecting appetite through their action on the higher centers in the brain. Because of their widespread abuse as stimulant drugs, however, the amphetamines (Benzedrine, Dexedrine) and methamphetamines (Desoxyn, Syndrox) were reclassified in 1971 to come under the provisions of the Drug Abuse Prevention and Control Act. Under these controls, which caused an 82 percent cutback in production quotas, prescription of these drugs for use in weight reduction fell off sharply, but they were replaced in part by substitute drugs—all chemically and pharmacologically related to the amphetamines, according to the FDA.

A panel of medical consultants advised the FDA in 1972 that the value of amphetamine-related diet drugs was "clinically trivial" and, in view of their potential for abuse, such drugs should be brought under even tighter controls. The FDA proceeded along several fronts. Stricter labeling was required for these drugs to point up the limitations on their usefulness, as well as the risk of dependence. A second cut in the production of amphetamines was also authorized. Amphetamines and closely related substances in injectable form were prohibited altogether as unsafe because of high drug abuse potential.

At the same time, amphetamines in combination with other drugs (mostly tranquilizers and sedatives) were also banned. The FDA estimated that 72 percent of the drugs prescribed by physicians as appetite suppressants were combinations of amphetamines and other drugs. Yet an FDA review of drug studies submitted by pharmaceutical firms showed that the combinations were no more effective than amphetamines used alone.

All amphetamine-type drugs prescribed as diet pills were brought under control of the Justice Department's Drug Enforcement Administration in 1973. The action imposed limitations on sales of amphetamine substitutes, but did not place them in the same highly restricted category as the amphetamines.

A survey of 480 physicians, published in *The Journal of the American Medical Association* in July 1973, revealed that of the doctors questioned only one-third did not prescribe appetite suppressants. And of the two-thirds who did use these drugs, most appeared to be "selective in their choice and use of drugs." However, some authorities believe that prescription of these drugs is never justified. At Senate hearings in December 1972 it was asserted that pharmaceutical manufacturers find fat people very interesting "mainly because there are so many of them." Other witnesses remarked that the pills gave doctors an easy out in dealing with their many obese patients.

There is no doubt that amphetamine drugs and related prescription medications can be used to suppress the appetite temporarily. But an effective dose varies with different individuals, and side effects are common (see below). Tolerance to these drugs is easily acquired, and after a period of several weeks increased doses may be required for continued appetite suppression.

In one careful five-year study, it was shown that excellent results in weight reduction usually were obtained in the first month or two of treatment under a physician's guidance, whether or not drugs were used, and regardless of type of drug. Results in patients treated by diet alone compared favorably with results in patients treated with a combination of diet and amphetamine drugs. The outcome undoubtedly reflected, in both groups of patients, enthusiasm and willingness. The study also showed side effects—dry mouth, irritability, restlessness, insomnia, rapid heartbeat, lightheadedness—from the use of amphetamine drugs.

Although studies have shown some effectiveness of appetite suppressants in the initial period of dieting (four to six weeks), the advantage over dieting managed without any drugs is so small and lasts for so short a time, and the risks of dependency are so large, that most overweight people are well advised to begin their campaign without the aid of drugs. Even the limited success possible with diet pills can come at some risk to the drug user. In addition to the side effects listed above, the patient may experience a letdown feeling when the drugs are no longer taken. While the effectiveness of drugs in weight reduction falls off sharply with continued usage, the same cannot be said of the possibility of dependence. A dieter could often wind up a fat person who takes amphetamines after starting out simply a fat person.

In 1978 about 3.3 million prescriptions were written for amphetamines, all but some 10 to 20 percent prescribed for weight reduction. Because of continuing evidence of widespread abuse of amphetamines, the FDA proposed in July 1979 to withdraw its approval for use of the drug in treatment of overweight. The FDA noted that amphetamines "present a severe risk of dependence and harmful effects."

Although glandular disturbances are rarely the cause of obesity, hormones have often been prescribed over the years to treat overweight patients. One popular misconception—that obese people suffer from an underactive thyroid gland—led to the use of thyroid hormones for obesity. In sufficiently high doses these drugs can reduce body weight. However, the weight loss is from lean body mass—muscle and organ tissue—in addition to loss of body fat. And when therapy is discontinued, the weight is regained.

Even more important, treatment with thyroid hormone can have serious side effects, particularly on the heart. In 1978 the FDA acted to discourage the promotion and use of such drugs for obesity. The FDA required that thyroid and related drugs carry a prominent label about the danger for users. The label warns, in part, that large doses "may produce serious or even life-threatening manifestations of toxicity."

Another frequently touted hormone for weight loss —human chorionic gonadotropin, or HCG—does not appear to pose a toxicity problem. However, it does not appear to offer any benefit either. Secreted in the urine of pregnant women, HCG was first used in weight-reduction programs by the late Albert T. W. Simeons, M.D., in the 1950s. The Simeons regimen involved injections of HCG six days each week in combination with a diet of 500 calories. HCG was claimed to improve weight loss while appeasing hunger and promoting a feeling of well-being. Its use eventually spread to numerous "fat clinics" across the country, especially in California.

While HCG caught on in the commercial business of weight reduction, its reputation among medical scientists remained suspect. There was no plausible explanation for its supposed action, and a majority of the studies evaluating its efficacy failed to show any benefit beyond a placebo effect. However, virtually all of the HCG studies were criticized on one or more grounds. Most were considered too limited in size to produce conclusive findings. Others were faulted for not following the Simeons method precisely or for similar problems in methodology.

Then, in November 1976 *The Journal of the American Medical Association* published the findings of a relatively large-scale clinical trial of HCG conducted at the medical center of Lackland Air Force Base in Texas.

The research project involved 202 obese patients who were divided into two groups under carefully controlled conditions. Half received HCG injections as specified in the Simeons regimen, and half received injections of an inert substance. All were assigned the 500 calorie diet commonly prescribed with HCG shots. The results showed no significant difference in weight loss between the two groups. Patients lost similar amounts of weight on the strict 500 calorie diet whether they received HCG or placebo. Robert L. Young, M.D., the Air Force medical officer heading the project, reported that the research team "could not demonstrate by any objective indicator that HCG was beneficial in promoting weight loss, nor was there any significant difference in fat loss or body circumference measurements." Furthermore, Young reported, "There was no evidence that those receiving HCG were more satisfied with the program." While proponents of HCG still tout its benefits, none has offered any scientific evidence that HCG is anything more than an expensive—and profitable—placebo in the treatment of obesity.

Hormones are not included in over-the-counter preparations promoted as diet aids. Such OTC products frequently contain a grab bag of ingredients ranging from vitamins and bulk producers to caffeine, grapefruit extract, and cider vinegar. Two frequent ingredients in these concoctions are phenylpropanolamine, a drug with some pharmacological relationship to amphetamines, and benzocaine. Interestingly enough, phenylpropanolamine is used as a nasal decongestant in several cold preparations. Besides its action as a decongestant, phenylpropanolamine also has some stimulant effect. CU's medical consultants believe that phenylpropanolamine is much more appropriate for shrinking swollen nasal passages than for shrinking swollen waistlines.

Benzocaine is a local anesthetic used widely in sunburn preparations and first-aid products. The "rationale" behind its use in diet-aid capsules, tablets, and chewing gum is the theoretical anesthetic effect on either the lining of the mouth or the lining of the stomach, which—purportedly—would suppress the appetite. Despite the lack of any well-controlled studies to support this contention, optimistic dieters occasionally buy the idea—and the product.

In May 1979 the Associated Press reported that an FDA panel of experts found these two OTC drugs safe and effective for weight control. The FDA's only comment was that the panel report had not yet been "officially reviewed."A nonprofit periodical for medical professionals, *The Medical Letter,* noted in August 1979 that the FDA panel had based its findings of the drugs' effectiveness on studies that are not described or not published and whose authors are not identified. *The Medical Letter* concluded: "There is no good evidence that phenylpropanolamine, oral benzocaine or any other drug can help obese patients achieve long-term weight reduction." CU's medical consultants concur and suggest that overweight people not fritter their funds away on worthless "appetite suppressants."

Exercise and Machines

The battle of the bulge is also being fought in another arena, with mechanical and electrical devices arrayed in the home and in slenderizing salons, gymnasiums, and health clubs. Various devices may provide active exercise, passive exercise, vibration, or massage. Although these devices and the methods of using them differ, there is generally one common feature: They are promoted primarily in terms of girth reduction, as distinguished from weight reduction.

The direct value of exercise in weight reduction is easy to overestimate. But it does have a place in a well-rounded reducing program based primarily on diet. For purposes of dieting, active exercise can be defined most helpfully in terms of calorie expenditure—the number of calories used up in a given amount of time by means of a particular form of exercise. After a study of the relationship between physical activity and obesity in women, two physicians, Anna-Marie Chirico and Albert Stunkard, concluded: "The physical activity of so many obese women is so severely limited that even small increases might favorably alter caloric balance. Treatment of these women, then, might profitably encourage efforts at increasing their physical activity."

To this limited extent, then, there may be merit in appeals to the overweight by some exercise centers, so far as the claims concern swimming or other physical activities, including the use of devices that make various muscles work against weights or springs. The value of exercise in losing weight is not one of spot reducing, even when the use of certain muscles is emphasized. It is a matter of expending calories that the body will recover equally from all fatty tissue.

These are advantages of *active* exercise, in which physical effort is initiated and maintained by the overweight person. However, considerably less can be expected from the passive exercise provided by devices that do the exercise for you—power-driven exercise machines, rocking tables, vibrators, and other more fanciful electrical devices. Among the latter was the *Relax-A-Cizor,* a low-voltage electrical apparatus that promised to reduce girth by electrical stimulation of the muscles.

The theory behind the *Relax-A-Cizor* was that an overweight person's muscles are soft and flabby and that stimulating them to contract by means of electrical impulses improves their tone and causes them to shrink. The claims for the *Relax-A-Cizor,* so far as it can be learned, were never subjected to scientifically controlled tests. What's more, the underlying theory seems to belie the biological facts. The muscles of a fat person are not necessarily soft, but rather overlaid with fat. Further, it is an *unused* muscle that shrinks; repeated contraction of a muscle should, if anything, lead to its enlargement.

In 1970 a permanent injunction against the distribution of the *Relax-A-Cizor* was issued by a United States district court. After a trial at which the views of thirty-one medical authorities were presented, the device was declared to be dangerous to health, having the potential effect of inducing abnormal rhythms of the heart, as well as causing miscarriages and aggravating such conditions as hernia, ulcers, varicose veins, and epilepsy.

Motor-driven rowing machines or bicyclelike devices yield the benefits of exercise in proportion to the amount of effort that goes into the movements. If you merely relax on the machine and let it pull you through the motions, it may be soothing in the way a massage is soothing, and it may contribute slightly to improved muscle tone. If you really want exercise, however, it would seem more to the point to use a machine without a motor.

Perhaps the most common devices promoted for the overweight are vibrators—everything from elaborate tables, couches, chairs, and beds to cushions, belts, and small hand-held appliances at prices ranging from a few dollars to several hundred. The vibrations of some of the larger devices cause passive body movements by means of rhythmic, rocking motions. What value there is in such motions is not known, but it is incorrect to assert, as has been done, that forty-five minutes on a rocking table is equivalent to playing thirty-six holes of golf or riding ten miles at a canter. The motion can be relaxing and soothing for many people, but it cannot, in fact, have any real effect on overweight.

In most other devices the vibrations are faster and the movements smaller. Promoters of devices often claim that their products (usually in conjunction with a diet plan) will produce a "firmer, more graceful figure" and provide "exercise without effort" and "relief of tension and fatigue." Some make broader claims—relief of pain, easing the symptoms of arthritis, and relief of menstrual cramps, backaches, headaches, and high blood pressure. As a result, many promoters have been in trouble with the federal government, since such medical claims bring the devices under the regulations of the FDA.

All claims that vibrators are effective in promoting weight reduction or treating disease are probably false and misleading. But some of the less definite claims may have a certain basis in fact. Although comprehensive and controlled studies of the effect of vibrators on the human body have not been made, it is conceivable that the devices may produce effects similar to those provided by the classic massage technique. Massage has been used since ancient times to soothe tired painful joints and muscles and to induce relaxation. Massage causes a slight increase in surface blood flow and skin temperature.

However, this is far from saying that the use of a vibrating bed, pillow, abdominal belt, or other device will "tone up" muscles and reduce girth. Nor will massage (whether done by hand, vibrator device, or the mechanical rollers that pound the hips of people in television commercials) remove fat deposits under the skin. Testifying before a congressional subcommittee in 1957, S. W. Kalb, M.D., reported the results of a study he had made on the effects of massage on body girth. Six weeks of twice-weekly massage of an arm and a leg produced no significant decrease in girth when compared with the unmassaged arm and leg of the same patient. In test subjects who were simultaneously dieting, decrease in girth was approximately the same in both limbs.

In some cases the federal government has come to the aid of the gullible consumer. A hearing examiner for the U.S. Postal Service ruled in 1972 that the firm promoting *Wonder Belt* was guilty of false advertising when it claimed that its device was capable of making obese people lose weight. The Postal Service stopped payment of postal money orders for the belt, and would-be purchasers had their letters ordering the product returned to them. Prospective buyers had been taken in by claims that *Wonder Belt* would reduce the amount of fat around the user's midsection and would cause a weight loss even without a change in daily routine or reduction in caloric intake.

In recent years there has been a proliferation of wearable products promoted for weight reduction—so-called sauna shorts and belts, body wraps dipped in chemical solutions, and others. All are ineffective at best, and some are downright dangerous. Physicians have warned that body wraps can be hazardous for people suffering from diabetes or diseases of the arteries and veins of the legs.

CU's medical consultants believe there are no short-cuts to weight reduction and to weight control. Long-term weight control, even with careful medical supervision, has been achieved by only a minority of patients. In most cases, weight loss is maintained for no more than several months at a time. The shrunken fat cells in the obese dieter tend to fill out over and over again.

Almost invariably doomed to failure in the treatment

of overweight are crash diets for taking off pounds quickly. Indeed, most of the weight loss achieved in the first week or two *on any diet* is due to elimination of excess water. In order to lose one pound of fat, the dieter must eliminate 3,500 calories. For example, if current daily intake totals 2,700 calories, and this daily intake is lowered by 500 calories to 2,200 calories per day, weight loss theoretically should proceed at the rate of one pound per week—assuming all other variables remain stable. However, it is difficult to maintain constant levels of exercise; metabolic factors differ from person to person, and the amount of water retained by the body may vary from day to day. Therefore it is not unusual for someone on a calorie-restricted diet to lose weight in a highly irregular fashion, sometimes remaining at a plateau for weeks at a time.

The dieter can speed up weight loss, if desired, by increasing calorie expenditure through exercise. And over the long term, of course, the number of calories burned through regular exercise can total quite a few pounds. That exercise is self-defeating is one of the myths perpetuated by the sedentary obese. It is *not* true in most cases that physical activity increases food intake. However, it takes a considerable amount of exercise to match the effect of calorie restriction. For example, a vigorous squash racquets game with active play lasting thirty minutes may result in an expenditure of 300 calories. The same net calorie loss could be accomplished just by passing up a single serving of lemon meringue pie.

Some studies have demonstrated that a "self-help" group can be as effective in facilitating weight loss as even the most sympathetic physician. However, before beginning such a program, it's advisable to check with your physician to confirm that dieting is indeed necessary and would not be detrimental to health.

All the answers to the treatment of obesity are obviously not yet available. As of this writing, CU's medical consultants believe that the best results for the least cost to health and pocketbook can be obtained by long-term calorie restriction, regular and well-balanced meals, and moderate exercise. Fad diets, over-the-counter diet aids, drug therapy, and exercise gadgets can't reshape the overweight. For permanent results, obese people must change their life-styles—permanently.

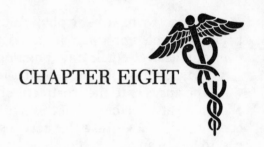

CHAPTER EIGHT

Chiropractors: Healers or Quacks?

In a voice charged with emotion, Joseph Janse, a chiropractor and president of the National College of Chiropractic, was addressing the hushed audience in the conference room.

"For me to stand here and exclaim or explain that I and my people, or those who preceded me, have never indulged in mishap or overclaim . . . would be dishonest. . . . I am not, and we are not, necessarily proud of those that we are responsible for, and have to live with. But I do hope . . . this workshop will not deny the people of my profession the privilege of progress and ethics."

As on many previous occasions, Janse was responding to a challenge to chiropractic. But this occasion in February 1975 was different from the rest.

The conference, a "Workshop on the Research Status of Spinal Manipulative Therapy," was taking place in Bethesda, Maryland, at the National Institutes of Health. Never before had chiropractors participated in an international scientific conference in the United States, much less at the NIH, one of the world's foremost medical and biological research organizations. Since 1895, in fact, chiropractic has largely rejected or ignored advances in medical science fostered by agencies like the NIH. In turn, many medical and government officials have generally branded chiropractic as "an unscientific cult" or "a significant hazard to the public." This time, however, the planning commission for the meeting—which was held in response to a Congressional mandate—included three chiropractors among its eight members.

The arrival of chiropractic in such a prestigious stronghold of science marked an important development that appeared to lend support to the chiropractor's demand for general recognition as a legitimate practitioner of the healing arts.

Despite opposition from organized medicine and the U.S. Public Health Service, chiropractors in 1973 won the right to render some services under both Medicare and Medicaid. Soon after, they achieved licensure in Louisiana and Mississippi, the last two holdouts among the fifty states. (The same period saw similar chiropractic gains in Canada.)

The crowning triumph for American chiropractors came in August 1974, when the U.S. Commissioner of Education recognized an accrediting agency for chiropractic colleges. This meant that colleges accredited by the Council on Chiropractic Education would have official national standing. Previously, degrees conferred by such institutions—for example, the Doctor of Chiropractic degree (D.C.)—were listed as "spurious" by the

U.S. Office of Education. Recognition also meant that accredited chiropractic schools would be eligible for financial assistance under federal funding programs.

Chiropractic, in short, has made undeniable progress in professional status and access to government-funded programs. Whether those gains mean equivalent progress for health care, however, is another question. In Consumers Union's view, the answer depends on whether chiropractic is a valid method of treatment or, as its critics contend, a form of quackery.

To explore that question, in 1975 CU studied the claims and practices of the profession to determine what chiropractic is and what potential benefit or harm a patient might experience. This chapter is based on a six-month investigation that included an extensive review of chiropractic and medical literature, as well as the findings of pertinent national, state, and provincial government studies conducted in the United States and Canada during the last decade or so. CU visited three chiropractic colleges—Palmer, National, and Canadian Memorial—and also interviewed officials of the principal chiropractic associations, whose memberships at that time included virtually all of the fifteen thousand chiropractors in active practice in the United States and some fourteen hundred chiropractors in Canada. CU also conducted interviews with American Medical Association representatives and with medical practitioners in orthopedics, physical medicine, neurosurgery, radiology, and other specialties. In the interest of objectivity, the assistance of CU's medical consultants was sought only for clarifying medical terminology or practices.

Chiropractic, which literally means "done by hand," originates from the theories of Daniel David Palmer, a tradesman who operated a "magnetic healing" studio in Davenport, Iowa, late in the nineteenth century. According to Palmer's writings, one of the passions of his life had been to discover the ultimate cause of disease—why one person should be ill while another person, "eating at the same table, working in the same shop," was spared illness. "This question," according to Palmer, "had worried thousands for centuries and was answered in September 1895."

The answer occurred to him, wrote Palmer, after treating a janitor he claimed was deaf. Palmer alleged that he restored the man's hearing by adjusting one of his vertebrae, the bony segments of the spine.

Apparently unaware that the nerves of hearing are entirely in the skull, Palmer theorized that he had relieved pressure on a spinal nerve that affected hearing. Adjusting the vertebrae, he decided, had removed interference with the nerve supply and thereby allowed the body's "Innate Intelligence" to effect a cure. Innate Intelligence, according to Palmer, was the "Soul, Spirit or Spark of Life," which he believed expressed itself through the nervous system to control the healing process. By supposedly impeding that expression, misaligned vertebrae were judged by Palmer as the cause of most disease.

In 1895 Palmer's emphasis on the spine raised fewer eyebrows among medical practitioners than it does today. Louis Pasteur had only recently demonstrated the plausibility of the germ theory of disease. And little more than a generation separated Palmer from many eminent physicians who had considered the spine to be the seat of innumerable human ills. It had been a common practice, in fact, to apply leeches, irritants, or even hot irons to tender sites along the spine as a treatment for various disorders. By the end of the nineteenth century, however, such practices had waned. The scientific revolution that would extend the boundaries of medicine in the twentieth century had already begun.

Osteopathy, which emerged a few years before chiropractic, adapted to the change. While retaining a separate identity—in part because of its use of manipulative therapy and its emphasis on the muscles and skeletal system—osteopathy gradually adopted the concepts and practices of orthodox medical science as well. Osteopathic students now receive training similar to that of medical students and earn a Doctor of Osteopathy (D.O.) degree. In contrast, chiropractic maintained its allegiance to the nineteenth-century focus on the spine.

Some chiropractors still cling strictly to Palmer's theory that misalignments of the vertebrae—or "subluxations"—are the principal cause of disease. Such practitioners tend to advertise that chiropractic is crucial to good health. For instance, in 1974 one ad called vertebral subluxation "a killer of millions of people yearly." In the main, however, chiropractic recognizes other factors in illness. It does tend to assign bacteria and viruses a back seat, but it no longer ignores their existence. Essentially, it has modified Palmer's theories to accommodate some basic scientific realities. Modern chiropractic, for example, agrees with medicine that germs are factors in disease and that the body has inherent defense mechanisms against them. However, chiropractic stresses that *mechanical* disturbances of the nervous system are what impair the body's defenses. According to this theory, minor "off-centerings" of the vertebrae or pelvis might disturb nerve function and lower the body's resistance to germs. Structural misalignments, say chiropractors, may also disturb nerve impulses to the visceral organs, allegedly causing or aggravating such illnesses as heart disease, stomach ulcers, and diabetes.

"While many factors impair man's health, disturbances of the nervous system are among the most important," asserts the American Chiropractic Association. According to the ACA, almost anything can cause a mechanical subluxation that might trigger nerve disturbances: gravitational strain, asymmetrical activities and efforts, developmental defects, or other mechanical, chemical, or psychic irritations. "Once produced," claims the association, "the lesion becomes a focus of sustained pathological irritation." While Palmer's theory of disease has been modified, the primary chiropractic treatment for all human illness remains the same as in 1895: spinal adjustment.

Chiropractic adjustment is a specific form of spinal manipulation. The technique, which is also used occasionally by osteopaths, physical therapists, and some medical doctors, is distinguished by the suddenness or speed of the maneuver, which prevents any control by the patient. By comparison, a patient can voluntarily resist—and therefore control—a manipulation when the therapist does it slowly or rythmically. If there is pain, for example, the patient can physically prevent further movement or advise the therapist accordingly. The latter technique, which is generally called mobilization, is the most common type of joint manipulation used by physical therapists.

In contrast, chiropractors emphasize the sudden maneuver, which they call a dynamic thrust. It may be done gently or forcefully, but always with a quick movement. The maneuver often produces a clicklike sound in the manipulated joint.

Those medical and osteopathic practitioners who use this technique say that it is sometimes effective for treating certain joint abnormalities or pain originating in the back or neck. There is disagreement among them, however, about what conditions it helps and exactly how it does so.

One prominent theory is that the manipulation essentially restores joint mobility, including a measure of "joint play" that isn't apparent in voluntary movements. Another is that the technique may displace a small fragment of a spinal disk that may be pressing against adjacent tissue. Others suggest that the sudden force may stretch a contracted muscle or tear adhesions, possibly relieving a local pain-causing spasm. Some manipulators subscribe to one theory while others believe several are possible. As yet, there's no proof that any of these theories are correct.

The chiropractic explanation is that the maneuver corrects subluxations. The current chiropractic definition of subluxation is so broad, however, that it takes in virtually any mechanical or functional derangement of the spine—or, as one speaker at the NIH workshop put it, "any variance from the normalcy of a newborn child." As a result, the chiropractic view does not reject any of the other theories. A locked joint or offending disk fragment would simply be labeled a subluxation.

Thus, most manipulators believe that their action affects some local condition, whatever it may be. The real quarrel arises when chiropractors claim that their manipulation also influences the nervous system and helps prevent or cure disease, an issue we will discuss later in this chapter.

Despite chiropractic's origin and all-embracing theory of disease, many people tend to view chiropractors as specialists in muscle or joint problems, particularly those of the back. Part of the reason, of course, is that chiropractic manipulation focuses on the spine. Whatever its ultimate intent, the therapy involves direct, physical action on the back. So people may conclude that that's what the treatment is for.

But there are other reasons as well for this traditional association. For one thing, the medical contemporary of the early chiropractor gave little priority to back ailments. The new science of bacteriology held immense promise for treating otherwise fatal illnesses, as did other developments in diagnosis and in surgery. Hence, medical efforts in the first third of this century focused on infectious disease and similarly urgent problems. Backaches could wait. Not until the 1930s did the medical profession start paying much attention to physical medicine and rehabilitation. In the interim, chiropractic seemed to offer hope in an area that medicine had largely ignored.

Even today, many physicians find little satisfaction in treating back ailments. Chronic pain may often be influenced by psychological problems or by physical habits that patients are unable or unwilling to change. Exact diagnosis can be elusive and expensive, and follow-up treatment can be time-consuming for the doctor. Specialists in physical medicine and orthopedics interviewed by CU asserted that, too often, treatment by some physicians simply has meant prescribing a painkiller, muscle relaxant, or tranquilizer rather than taking the time and effort that such ailments might demand.

Chiropractors, meanwhile, have usually been ready and willing to see patients repeatedly and to provide active treatment—manipulation, exercise programs, heat application, and the like. In CU's opinion, such accommodation has probably reinforced the belief that chiropractors specialize in back ailments. Indeed, a survey conducted in 1967 by the University of Kentucky College of Medicine revealed that most of the people in the study who visited chiropractors believed that a chiropractor has more specialized training in musculoskeletal back and joint problems than a physician has. Actually, chiropractors usually have more training than medical doctors in only one area: manipulative therapy.

Chiropractors who belong to the International Chiropractors Association often confine their treatment solely to manipulation. Besides spinal adjustment, treatment may include various "soft-tissue" manipulations, such as massaging muscles or applying sustained pressure to ligaments. But the basic approach is "hands only."

The majority of chiropractors, however, use a variety

of treatment techniques. The scope generally depends on what's permitted by state or provincial law. Chiropractors may not practice surgery or prescribe medications. But many jurisdictions allow them to use physiotherapy and to recommend various nutritional supplements, such as vitamins and minerals.

The types of treatment are often similar to some used by physicians or physical therapists (although the purpose of application may not always be the same). In addition to exercise programs, such measures may include the use of a brace or cast, whirlpool baths, hot or cold packs, ultrasound, diathermy, and other devices.

Chiropractic, in short, is seldom limited to spinal adjustment alone. Chiropractors often can, and do, make use of common measures for treating muscle or joint complaints. And some limit their practice almost exclusively to such complaints, frankly dismissing Palmer's disease theory as "cultism" or "chiroquackery."

An undetermined number also try to cooperate with local physicians, referring to them patients who appear to need medical care and occasionally receiving a referral in turn. In April 1975, for instance, *Medical Economics,* a magazine distributed to physicians, reported the response of more than one thousand office-based M.D.s to a survey it conducted of referral relationships with chiropractors. More than 20 percent of the physicians responding to the survey stated that they received some referrals from chiropractors. Also 5 percent of the respondents said they sometimes referred patients to chiropractors.

On the basis of CU's 1975 investigation, however, such instances of cooperation, or of chiropractic willingness to limit its scope of practice, tended to be the exception rather than the rule. Chiropractic officials and educators invariably told CU that the chiropractor's role was that of a primary physician, not a muscle-and-joint practitioner. They emphasized that chiropractors should serve as one of the "portals of entry" to the health-care system, functioning essentially as family doctors and referring patients, when appropriate, to other health professions.

Such a role assumes that chiropractors, despite much less diagnostic training than M.D.s or D.O.s, will recognize when to treat a patient and when to refer one to a physician. It's on this point—and on the question of scientific validity—that chiropractic clashes most seriously with organized medicine.

For years, chiropractors have argued that medical or scientific opposition to chiropractic is largely a business quarrel. According to the charge, organized medicine is a monopoly concerned primarily with aggrandizement of physicians, and the American Medical Association is just trying to keep out the competition. The book *Chiropractic: A Modern Way to Health,* which was recommended to CU by chiropractic officials, typically points the accusing finger at the AMA: ". . . the AMA is a private group of men and women with a common private business interest, namely the practice of medicine," according to the author, Julius Dintenfass, D.C., a charter member of the New York State Board of Chiropractic Examiners. "Despite their vaunted concern for the public health and welfare, the medical sachems act toward chiropractic as any collection of businessmen being threatened by a rival concern which seems to have the kind of merchandise that customers prefer."

When CU discussed that allegation with the chiropractic officials, we expected to find wide agreement with it. We didn't. "It's not true," said Richard C. Schafer, D.C., director of public affairs for the American Chiropractic Association, in an interview with CU. "The average medical doctor has more patients than he can handle," Schafer said. "They're not afraid of competition."

Why, then, has organized medicine for so many years opposed chiropractic? CU got several answers from AMA representatives and other critics. They involved charges of inferior education and training, rejection of medical science, and abuses or hazards arising from the practice of chiropractic. Since those allegations have serious implications for patient care and safety, CU investigated them in detail.

There is virtually no denial that educational standards for chiropractors in the past were often little short of appalling. As late as 1942, according to *Medical Economics,* it was still possible to get the mail-order Doctor of Chiropractic degree from a Chicago college for $127.50.

Although standards did improve, glaring deficiencies were apparent until fairly recently. The scope of the problem was outlined in a thorough evaluation of chiropractic schools conducted in 1964 by Dewey Anderson, Ph.D., who was at that time the director of education for the ACA. Some of the inadequacies that were mentioned in Anderson's 1964 report were: "Too many instructors teaching the basic sciences without having had any advanced or graduate training in these sciences. Too many instructors not trained or qualified as teachers nor masters of their fields, resulting in slavish devotion to textbook teaching and instruction considerably below the level of post-college professional education."

The academic credentials of the students, Anderson noted, were similarly deficient: "One of the most serious handicaps . . . is that of trying to teach at the post-college professional level students who for the most part have not gone beyond high school, and who in high school were not in the upper half of their classes. For many of them a professional college course is too difficult to master." The result, said Anderson, was to downgrade instruction so that students could pass the courses.

A comprehensive study of chiropractic conducted in 1965 for the Government of Quebec reached similar conclusions. Student admission requirements were termed "too liberal, and inadequate," and the training required of teachers was judged "definitely inferior" to that demanded either by medical schools or by university science departments. "A great number of these teachers are chiropractors who have received training in basic sciences of very little value," said the Quebec study.

Landmark studies of chiropractic by the U.S. Department of Health, Education, and Welfare in 1968 and Ontario's Committee on the Healing Arts in 1970 expressed similarly critical findings. In addition to poorly qualified teachers, inferior basic science courses, and notably low admission requirements, both reports criticized the lack of emphasis on research. The HEW report also noted the absence of inpatient hospital training and a poor ratio of faculty to students. At the time of the HEW study, chiropractic schools averaged about one faculty member for each nineteen students, compared with 1 per 1.7 students in medical schools. (Both figures included part-time instructors with administrative duties or outside practices.)

"The scope and quality of chiropractic education do not prepare the practitioner to make an adequate diagnosis and provide appropriate treatment," the HEW report concluded. The Ontario committee endorsed the HEW findings on education and judged the chiropractor's diagnostic ability as "very limited at best."

A study conducted for the State of Wisconsin in 1972 found conditions largely unchanged. While commending the "sincerity and dedication" of both students and faculty, the Wisconsin study committee concluded that "the deficiencies are too pervasive to permit an adequate educational experience."

Since the early 1970s, chiropractic schools generally have sought to raise their educational standards. This was evident at the colleges CU visited in 1974–75. They still required only a "C" average for admission, but entering students had to have two years of college or the equivalent, including courses in biology and chemistry. Actually, about half of the entrants at National College of Chiropractic in Lombard, Illinois, and at Canadian Memorial College of Chiropractic in Toronto already had college degrees.

The change in the academic background of students was perhaps most dramatic at Palmer College of Chiropractic in Davenport, Iowa, which is by far the world's largest chiropractic school (Palmer trains about one-third of all chiropractors). Its January 1975 enrollment still included about 550 students whose previous education was limited to high school or an equivalency program. Virtually all were seniors scheduled to graduate that year, however. The rest of Palmer's approximately 2,100 students had one or more years of college; 416 of them held college degrees.

Academic requirements for faculty members have also been upgraded. Increasingly, instructors in basic science subjects must have recognized qualifications in their disciplines, and the colleges are giving preference to candidates with graduate degrees.

Insistence on advanced qualifications tended to be most pronounced at National College. Instructors in basic sciences generally had to have a graduate degree in their specialty, and the college said it would not hire a teacher with only a master's degree unless the candidate's department already included a Ph.D. A doctor of chiropractic degree was still acceptable, though, for instructors in chiropractic or clinical courses.

In short, chiropractors were no longer teaching all subjects. And the colleges have also narrowed the ratio of faculty to students. Canadian Memorial, for example, had roughly one teacher for every eight students in 1975. Instructors were still spread fairly thin at Palmer, with one per thirty students. But that was an improvement over its 1-to-45 ratio of a few years earlier. Library facilities have also been expanded, and National College, for one, initiated a modest research project with a federal agency.

Despite improvements in other areas, education in diagnosis remains a stepchild—especially in comparison with training received by physicians. Part of the problem is historical. Traditionally, chiropractors believed it wasn't important to "name" a disease. The important thing was to find and correct the subluxation allegedly causing it. It made little difference, for example, if a liver disorder involved congestion, cirrhosis, or cancer; the object was to relieve nervous-system disturbances that were supposedly responsible for the disorder.

Accordingly, that approach placed little or no emphasis on making a differential diagnosis—that is, one that considers possible causes of a patient's symptoms and establishes probable as well as alternative diagnoses. While differential diagnosis is fundamental in the practice of medicine, chiropractors generally shunned it, preferring to call their approach "spinal analysis" rather than diagnosis. Even today, some practitioners insist that medical diagnosis is out of place in chiropractic.

"It is a trap for the unwary in this profession," wrote William D. Harper, D.C., president of Texas Chiropractic College, in 1975 in *The Digest of Chiropractic Economics.* "We waste too much time in our curriculum on medical diagnosis."

Many chiropractic officials and educators disagree with that sentiment, however. And diagnostic training has become an integral part of the curriculum at most chiropractic colleges. Yet many of the people teaching diagnosis are the very same chiropractors who were trained in the 1960s and earlier, when educational standards—and attitudes toward diagnosis—were far from ideal. These instructors, moreover, labor under a burden common to all chiropractors—the lack of inpatient hospital training.

"The medical doctor has the benefit of patient exposure that we do not have," noted Andries M. Kleynhans, D.C., director of clinical sciences at National College. Because of the lack of chiropractic hospitals, chiropractors seldom see or treat diseases that the medical doctor does. That gap, Kleynhans told CU, places chiropractors at a disadvantage in their diagnostic training.

In addition, chiropractors cannot use many of the sophisticated diagnostic techniques available to the physician. This is true even for some major diagnostic aids involving the spine. A herniated spinal disk, for example, isn't visible on a simple X ray. If it's necessary to confirm the disk protrusion, a physician may order a myelogram, an X-ray technique that involves injecting an opaque dye into the space surrounding the spinal cord. Chiropractors are neither trained to interpret myelograms nor permitted to perform them.

Nor do they have the benefit of the more extensive education and training required of physicians. In contrast to the chiropractor's two years of college (now) and four years of professional school, the physician must have four years of college, four years of medical school, and usually three or more years of hospital residency. Moreover, the physician's subsequent affiliation with a hospital provides a center for continuing education. At the hospital, the physician's medical knowledge is reinforced and expanded through conferences, discussions, and association with colleagues, as well as through experiences with patients. Chiropractors, in comparison, generally work alone.

Clearly, the scope, quality, and length of chiropractic education cannot provide the depth of diagnostic training a physician receives. Even more fundamental, however, is the validity of what the chiropractor learns. If it's unsound, more training might only compound the error. The crucial question, therefore, is whether chiropractic theory is true or false.

The belief that minor interference with the spinal nerves can cause or aggravate disease is the cornerstone of chiropractic theory. It is also the focus of scientific objections. A few anatomical facts may help to explain why.

There are twenty-six pairs of nerves that exit from mobile segments of the spine. They are the only part of the nervous system conceivably accessible to manipulation. Twelve pairs of cranial nerves, which exit through openings in the base of the skull and bypass the spine, are out of reach of manipulation. So, too, are five pairs exiting from the sacrum, a solid bone formed by the fusion of five vertebrae in the lower spine. The spinal cord (which is surrounded by spinal fluid as well as by protective layers of tissue) and the brain itself—with all its interconnecting nerve pathways—are also out of reach.

Thus, the chiropractor's action is exerted on only a limited part of the nervous system. It excludes, for example, the nerves of sight, hearing, taste, and smell, and the entire parasympathetic nervous system. The latter, along with the sympathetic nervous system, form the balancing halves of the autonomic, or "involuntary," nervous system, which serves the vital organs.

Scientists, of course, accept the importance of the nervous system in body functions. What they reject is the assertion that manipulation directed at a limited part of this intricate system can prevent or cure disease. In the first place, there's no scientific evidence that minor off-centerings of the vertebrae impinge on spinal nerves. One study in 1973, which tested fresh cadaver spines, suggested that impingement does not occur even when the spine is twisted into extreme positions or abnormal forces are applied to the vertebrae. Second, if such a partial block could occur, its effect would be nil. Research by neurophysiologists shows that a nerve impulse travels more slowly in a zone of partial compression but resumes its flow immediately thereafter. The impulse transmitted is normal in all respects. What is perhaps hardest for scientists to accept, though, is chiropractic's singular concept of the nervous system itself.

According to that view, the nervous system is the overall master of all body functions, regulating everything from major organs to intricate cellular activities. A typical statement of this concept appears in the pamphlet "How Chiropractic Heals," one of many such pamphlets for patients distributed by chiropractors. "None of the body functions 'just happen,'" said the pamphlet. "Your heart doesn't just happen to beat. Your lungs don't just happen to inhale and exhale. Your stomach doesn't just happen to digest your dinner. *All* doctors know that your brain and nerve system coordinate these functions which make for life instead of death, health instead of sickness."

Actually, all doctors know no such thing. The heart just *does* happen to beat. It will beat for a period of time even if removed from the body and cut off from all nerve impulses, so long as it's surrounded by a nutrient fluid. Transplanted, it is capable of sustaining life in another human being without any immediate connection to the brain, spinal cord, or other nerve tissue. The heart has an intrinsic rhythm of its own and thus can function automatically.

Similarly, the stomach digests automatically. There are inherent processes that govern the functions of organs as important as the heart, stomach, intestines, blood vessels, and the like. Their function doesn't depend entirely on the nervous system. A paraplegic woman, for example, may conceive, carry her pregnancy to term, and give birth to a normal baby—despite severe injury to her spinal cord. Except for bladder and bowel problems, internal organs of a quadriplegic still continue to function, even though the spinal nerves are useless from the neck down. In short, life goes on—despite even massive "interference" with nerve impulses. That doesn't mean the spinal nerves aren't important. But their importance doesn't render other fundamental life processes trivial.

The immunological defense system, for instance, can work independently of nerve impulses. Artificially cultured white blood cells will continue to engulf germs even though entirely divorced from nerve influence. At the cellular level, to which chiropractic claims to extend, the same autonomy has been documented. Molecular research has become so precise that it can sometimes pinpoint which portion of a molecule is responsible for a particular disease. These biochemical life processes are fundamental—and completely independent of the nervous system.

Not a single scientific study in the eighty-five-year existence of chiropractic or the entire history of medicine shows that manipulation can affect any of these basic life processes. But a vast amount of evidence suggests it cannot.

In 1895 neither Palmer nor his contemporaries could foresee that research. Today, however, there's no excuse for ignoring it. Unless most medical research in the twentieth century is wrong, Palmer's disease theory belongs in the pages of nineteenth-century history, along with bleeding, purging, and other blind alleys of medicine.

When chiropractic theory is put into practice, its efforts can sometimes border on the ludicrous. Several chiropractic pamphlets that have been used in Canada, for example, tout spinal manipulation as a cure for childhood bed-wetting. Actually, the nerves to the bladder emerge from the rigid bone of the sacrum. There is no way to manipulate them. Further, a true nerve defect would cause constant bladder problems, not just bed-wetting.

Spinal manipulation is also promoted frequently for patients with high blood pressure. A typical pamphlet obtained from the sales department at Palmer College suggests that the ailment may be treated through "proper adjustment by hand." While the basic causes of high blood pressure in most patients are still unknown, the portion of the nervous system involved in lowering blood pressure is well identified—the parasympathetic nervous system. It is fed by the cranial and sacral nerves, and, as noted earlier, is entirely inaccessible to manipulation.

"Eye Trouble," another pamphlet from Palmer, suggests that manipulation may be applicable to some eye problems. Yet the optic nerves are completely self-contained in the skull. There is no conceivable way to reach them manually. Other pamphlets obtained from Palmer tout manipulation for conditions ranging from acne and appendicitis to stomach trouble and tonsillitis. There isn't a shred of scientific evidence showing that those ailments respond to manipulation.

Such unproved claims have bedeviled some chiropractors for years. In an August 1974 letter, Herbert W. E. Poinsett, a Florida chiropractor, took the ACA to task for one of its pamphlets. "The new ACA tract on the kidneys is a disgrace to this profession," wrote Poinsett. "The statement, 'Your doctor of chiropractic treats many kidney disorders,' is pure nonsense! I ask you, what disorders?

"Does chiropractic treat the following successfully? Neoplasms, tumors of the adrenal gland, calculi, hydronephrosis, tuberculosis, nonspecific infections. . . . Are you telling the people that we can treat such pathologies? If you are, then we deserve the title of quack and cultists!"

"Many within the profession, I'm sure, may agree with your comments," an ACA official replied. However, he noted, others might want to utilize the tract in their practices. "This tract, in one version or another, has been a stock item for over forty years and has been redesigned to meet the sustained needs of the interested membership."

Most chiropractic officials interviewed by CU frankly admitted the problem of over-claiming. "We as a profession have claimed too much without valid proof," said Donald C. Sutherland, D.C., executive director of the Canadian Chiropractic Association. He indicated that the Canadian organization was actively trying to limit chiropractic's scope of practice. Neither in Canada nor in the United States, however, did CU find concrete evidence that abuses in the field were abating.

At the Sherman College of Chiropractic in Spartanburg, South Carolina, for example, the criteria for accepting a patient were liberal indeed. According to an editorial by Douglas Gates, a dean of the college, requirements for a "chiropractic case" were threefold: Does the patient have a spinal column? Does the patient have a nervous system? Is the patient alive?

For some chiropractors, economics probably plays a large part in the range of illnesses treated. A limited scope of practice can often mean fewer patients. And those who confine themselves to musculoskeletal problems—sprains, strains, and back or neck ailments—tend to cut their income potential.

According to the ACA, in 1974 United States chiropractors earned an average annual income of about $31,000. Canadian practitioners averaged roughly the same. Often contributing to the attainment of that income are various practice-building organizations that seem to abound within the profession.

Among the oldest of such groups is the Parker Chiropractic Research Foundation, which has offered a comprehensive, hard-sell approach for attracting patients and keeping them coming back. Since the 1950s, several thousand chiropractors or their assistants have attended the Parker courses. Encouraging practitioners to advertise, Parker has stressed the use of a Chiropractic Research Chart and a "nerve" chart. The former lists numerous disorders purportedly helped by chiropractic treatment and gives the percentage of "success" for each. The nerve chart shows a picture of the spine and specifies the diseases supposedly caused by misalignments at each level. Neither chart has any scientific validity or any acceptable evidence to support its claims. Because of such advertising, the Canadian Chiropractic Association has refused to release its mailing list to the Parker organization.

Another of the most successful practice builders is Clinic Masters, which has claimed a membership of about 12 percent of all United States and Canadian chiropractors in active practice. According to its membership contract, a chiropractor who "desires to have the Clinic Masters System revealed to him" must agree to pay $10,000 and not "divulge or share, directly or indirectly," any portion of the system with anyone other than a Clinic Masters client.

Clinic Masters has taught a variety of specific income-building techniques, promoting the idea that higher income means greater service to patients. Some ways of providing such service have included multiple billing, which means charging for each spinal adjustment or other unit of treatment rather than accepting a flat office fee; a "case basis" approach, which involves charging by the case (like a surgeon) rather than by number of visits; and "intensive day care," which adds room or ward fees to the bill.

In recognition of their "service to humanity," Clinic Masters clients have earned membership ranks in one of twelve clubs. The lowest was the Leviathan club, for those earning $4,000 to $8,000 a month. The highest was the Purple & White Medallion club, which was added for members earning $50,000 or more a month.

According to the major chiropractic associations, none of the billing practices mentioned above is considered "a reasonable and customary procedure" in the profession. But criticism has been stifled somewhat by Clinic Masters' threat to sue those whose remarks it judged to be libelous. It offered a $10,000 reward to anyone who was first to report and substantiate "disparaging statements about Clinic Masters" that led to a successful lawsuit.

Despite the excesses of some practitioners and chiropractic's rejection of science, the profession nevertheless maintains that it offers an important health service. And each year more than 5 million men, women, and children obtain chiropractic treatment in the United States and Canada. Many of these patients sincerely believe that chiropractors help them, that these practitioners are more than common quacks. But how many patients actually benefit from chiropractic treatment? And what risks do they face in the process?

Years ago some surgeons thought they had developed a promising cure for angina pectoris, the chest pains associated with coronary heart disease. Tying off an artery in the chest appeared to offer relief. The cure was short-lived, however. Subsequent research showed that a sham operation, consisting of just a superficial incision on the chest wall, was equally successful.

That experiment, like countless others, demonstrated the broad influence of the "placebo effect," a reaction to an inert medication or procedure that results in improvement or cure of symptoms. Because of it, a sham operation may ease anginal pain or, similarly, a dummy pill may relieve the nausea of pregnancy.

It matters little whether the treatment is surgery, drugs, manipulation, or incantations. The key factors in the placebo effect are the patient's confidence in the healer and the healer's faith in the therapy—especially when that faith is communicated to the patient.

Throughout much of medical history, the placebo effect was frequently all any healer could offer. Indeed, a patient was often fortunate if the actual treatment was of psychological value, or even merely worthless, rather than harmful or fatal. Today, despite all the acumen and paraphernalia of modern medicine, such psychological effects are still an important factor in therapy. And they frequently account for some of the benefits obtained from the most skilled of physicians. Such effects also explain, in part, why chiropractors can sometimes help people.

Physicians have long recognized the potent psychological effect of the "laying on of hands." Chiropractors at the National Institutes of Health conference in February 1975 also acknowledged its role in treatment. In fact, one prominent chiropractor, Scott Haldeman of Vancouver, British Columbia, felt that such placebo effects should be considered an advantage of manipulation.

"Clinicians who practice spinal manipulations often become very defensive when their detractors derisively state that all results can be explained on the basis of psychological effects," Haldeman said. "However, there are very few therapies that have the advantages of laying on of hands, relaxing tense muscles, causing a sensation in the area of pain, the click or pop of the adjustment, and a clinician who has complete confidence in his therapy. It is a pity that this possibility has been considered a criticism of the therapeutic procedure instead of one of its advantages."

Numerous studies show that placebo treatment in many disorders helps about one-third of patients. Temporary relief of pain or other symptoms has been demonstrated, for example, in arthritis, hay fever, headache, cough, high blood pressure, peptic ulcer, and even cancer.

The psychological aspects of many disorders also work to the healer's advantage. According to CU's interviews with specialists in internal medicine, one-third to one-half of the complaints patients present in routine office visits either do not arise from organic disease or have obvious psychological components. Hence, treatment offering some psychological benefit can often be helpful. A sympathetic ear for the patient's complaints or firm, authoritative reassurance that no serious disease is involved can prove therapeutic in itself.

One of the most important factors, suggested a physician at the NIH conference, is that patients are relieved of the responsibility for their illness and suffering when they hand that burden over to the healer. "That silent act," he asserted, "is probably . . . as important as anything else that goes on, and often many of the things that we do after that point we get by with rather than being effective with."

Beyond psychological influences in treatment, there are also the recuperative powers of the body itself. Medical scientists estimate that about two-thirds of human illnesses are self-limiting. Regardless of what type of outside intervention or treatment is used, the patients eventually get well on their own.

Even some chronic disorders, such as rheumatoid arthritis and multiple sclerosis, have spontaneous remissions. The symptoms may disappear, regardless of treatment, for months or more, affording temporary or, at times, long-term relief. If the patient happens to be under treatment at the time, the practitioner and the type of therapy may get credit for such relief.

Most back problems will also resolve themselves. Several studies show that about 60 percent of patients with back pain get well within three weeks and at least 90 percent recover within two months—regardless of the type of treatment received. Only about 2 percent eventually undergo surgery, usually for serious bone or disk problems.

Although physicians and chiropractors emphasize different methods of treatment for patients with common back problems, a study published in 1974 comparing both groups showed essentially no difference in the outcome of therapy. Both the physicians and the chiropractors achieved satisfactory results with more than

90 percent of patients suffering from back or neck ailments, according to the study, which was conducted by researchers at the University of Utah College of Medicine.

Perhaps the most interesting part of the study was the reaction of patients to their respective practitioners. The chiropractic patients were significantly more satisfied with the explanations they received about their problems and the degree to which they were made to feel welcome. Reporting their findings in *The Lancet*, a British medical journal, in June 1974, the authors stressed the implications of the patients' reactions: "On the basis of our study and others, it appears that the chiropractor may be more attuned to the total needs of the patient than is his medical counterpart. The chiropractor does not seem hurried. He uses language patients can understand. He gives them sympathy, and he is patient with them. He does not take a superior attitude toward them. In summary, it is an egalitarian relationship rather than a superordinate/subordinate relationship." Their findings, the authors concluded, "underscore the powerful potential for the doctor-patient relationship in effective treatment, whether in chiropractic or traditional medicine."

Many positive responses to chiropractic treatment undoubtedly stem from the doctor-patient relationship or the self-limiting nature of various illnesses. But some favorable results can be ascribed directly to manipulation itself. Government studies in the United States and Canada have judged manipulation to be a potentially useful technique for certain conditions, such as the loss of joint mobility. Research in manipulation is still meager, and controlled clinical studies are rare. But chiropractors and other practitioners who use manipulative therapy agree it can help some muscle or joint problems.

Treatment of tension headaches by massage, for example, is well recognized. Those headaches can stem from tense muscles in the neck, and massage may relieve symptoms. Some practitioners also report that a stiff joint in the neck may sometimes cause headache pain that can be treated by manipulation.

In general, back or neck pain that might arise from restricted movement in a spinal joint may respond to manipulation. Such pain is usually localized in the area of the joint. However, the pain may sometimes be referred to another part of the body, such as the chest. Referred pain may occasionally mimic the symptoms of other disorders, such as angina pectoris.

"Thus we find a perfectly reasonable basis in fact for the somewhat bizarre stories of miraculous cures by spinal manipulation," said John McM. Mennell, M.D., an authority on manipulative therapy. "Almost invariably the basis of these stories is that the patient has been told a diagnosis which he believes and remembers," wrote Mennell in his book *Back Pain.* "If his symptoms are then unrelieved by orthodox treatment, but are later cured by a manipulator, it is not surprising that the patient claims to have been cured of the visceral disease." Many chiropractors and other manipulators share Mennell's view.

There are, in short, a variety of possible reasons why patients may experience benefits from chiropractic treatment. That may not be all they experience, however. The Chiropractic Study Committee for the State of Wisconsin in 1972 underscored a critical issue surrounding chiropractic: "It is beyond question that substantial numbers of people believe themselves to have been helped by chiropractic treatment," said the committee report. "It is also beyond question that if they feel better, for whatever reason, they have, in some sense, been helped. There is, however, a balancing factor that screams to be considered. That, of course, is the potential hazard of treatment that ignores established scientific knowledge."

On the basis of CU's investigation, there are several major areas for concern. Since many human illnesses are self-resolving, any intervention by a practitioner should avoid exposing a patient to unnecessary risks. The maxim, as a medical aphorism puts it, is *primum non nocere:* "First of all, do no harm."

The ACA states that spinal manipulation is "a painless and safe procedure." But a review of chiropractic and medical literature by CU indicates that manipulation is not without hazard. The adverse effects reported range from minor sprains and soreness to serious complications and death. Serious complications included fracture, spinal disk rupture, paraplegia, and stroke. Chiropractors say that such catastrophic consequences of manipulation as stroke are relatively rare; and, indeed, CU's investigation uncovered only twelve documented cases of severe stroke from chiropractic manipulation from 1947 to 1976.

The exact incidence of injury is virtually impossible to determine, however. Unlike medical reports, none of the many chiropractic surveys and journals CU reviewed gave any statistics on complications. The only data are from isolated medical studies by a few physicians.

In an attempt to fill that gap, a study published in *Clinical Orthopaedics and Related Research* in 1971 reported the injuries from chiropractic manipulation recorded by one physician over a three-year period. The physician reported that 172 of the patients he examined in his practice had previously undergone chiropractic manipulation. Seven of those, or 4 percent, had suffered direct injuries, ranging from aggravation of pain to serious nerve damage. "Injury associated with spinal manipulation," the physician concluded, "appears more frequent than the present North American medical literature suggests."

Therapy often involves risks. The question is whether those risks are warranted. Many surgical procedures and drugs used in medical practice are hazardous. Accordingly, physicians will weigh such risks against the proved value of treatment so that patients will not be endangered unnecessarily. While an individual physician's judgment may be faulty, the emphasis of medicine on proved therapy tends to increase the average patient's chances of genuine therapeutic benefits for the risks taken.

If spinal manipulation were a proved form of universal therapy, there would be no reason to restrict it to muscle or joint disorders, even if it involved some risk. But as CU pointed out earlier, chiropractic use of manipulation in other illnesses contradicts much of the basic medical research of the twentieth century. In such applications, CU concludes, any risk of injury is unwarranted.

Unlike physicians, chiropractors receive no education or training in pharmacology and drug therapy. What they learn about drugs is often self-taught. That lack of scientific background or experience in drug therapy may well contribute to what CU views as a dangerous approach to drugs by many chiropractors. Specifically, it involves undermining the use of accepted drug therapies and espousing the use of unproved ones.

Various chiropractic pamphlets for the public employ direct scare tactics against drugs. Such titles as "Drug-Caused Diseases" and "Drugs—Dangerous Whether Pushed or Prescribed" are typical. One published by the ACA, "Beware of Overuse of Drugs," lists scores of possible adverse reactions to such drugs as antibiotics, oral contraceptives, and medicines for high blood pressure. The pamphlet then asserts that chiropractors use no drugs, "thus avoiding drug-induced illnesses and dangerous side effects often more serious than the condition being treated." There's no mention that some of those drugs may be life-saving for patients who need them.

A common tactic is to link drug-taking with drug abuse. "Don't be a pill popper," says the headline of an ad put out by the ACA. "Drugging your pain and your problems is not your answer to good health." According to the ad, "drugs and medications only mask the pain and dull the symptoms of a health problem."

The consequences of such advice can be tragic. These are typical of the cases CU has come across.

□Under chiropractic care, an elderly woman with high blood pressure was advised to stop medication. Her blood pressure rose sharply, and after a month she suffered a stroke.

□A diabetic patient gave up insulin on instruction of a chiropractor. An infection held in check by good control of the diabetes with insulin then spread and caused the patient's death.

□Parents of a six-year-old epileptic girl stopped anticonvulsive therapy on the advice of a chiropractor. Until then, the child had been doing well and was seizure-free. Without the medication, she had a prolonged seizure that resulted in brain damage and subsequent mental retardation.

Chiropractic antipathy to medication, however, appears limited to prescription drugs—which chiropractors may not legally prescribe. Other medications, such as vitamin preparations, are widely recommended and sold in chiropractic practice. In CU's opinion, that distinction can be a dangerous one. A substance is defined as a drug by its use, not by arbitrary categories. In medicine, a drug is any substance used as medication for a disease. Water prescribed for a dehydrated patient can be defined as a drug. Ordering vitamins for a deficiency disease is prescribing a drug.

For the patient's safety, any prescriber should have sufficient training to know when and why a specific drug is indicated. Chiropractors have no such training. In CU's view, a brief course in nutrition at a chiropractic school is no substitute for years of training in drug therapy. Yet chiropractors sometimes presume they can treat complex illnesses with vitamin pills.

Health Quackery

An article in the March 1975 issue of *The ACA Journal of Chiropractic,* for example, espoused high-dose vitamins for treating schizophrenia, a complex and sometimes crippling mental illness. The author noted that "there is a great deal of controversy" surrounding such treatment, but he concluded that "the megavitamin approach is a practical alternative" for treating schizophrenia. The approach, he said, "should be considered by chiropractic as an adjunct to spinal manipulation."

Indeed, there once was "a great deal of controversy" about megavitamin therapy for schizophrenia. But that was before several carefully controlled studies showed it to have no therapeutic benefit. On the contrary, the findings suggested potentially adverse effects, including longer hospitalization, increased need for other drugs, and poorer adjustment to home and community life after patients left the hospital. Overall, the treatment was judged inferior to a placebo. Thus, the chiropractic author is recommending that a complicated mental disorder be treated with a drug less effective than a dummy pill.

One of the worst dangers of chiropractic treatment, say its critics, is that it might divert the patient from seeking appropriate medical attention in time. The result, they contend, may have serious or even fatal consequences that might otherwise have been avoided.

Part of the problem is the confusing nature of back pain. Most patients who visit a chiropractor go initially because of back troubles. But back pain can arise from a variety of causes, ranging from a simple sprain to heart disease. It may be muscular or skeletal in origin, or a symptom of ulcers, cancer, or disorders of the uterus or ovaries. It can also be caused by diseases of the lungs, kidneys, liver, bladder, intestines, or other organs.

When a disorder of the internal organs is suspected, many chiropractors will refer the patient to a physician. But the chiropractors' limited diagnostic training presents a major handicap to early recognition of such illnesses. And some chiropractors will continue to treat a patient regardless of any diagnosis, apparently convinced by chiropractic theory that they are relieving the true cause of the disease. Meanwhile, with delay in proper treatment the illness may grow worse.

There is relatively little information available about the type or frequency of serious consequences resulting from such delays. According to American Medical Association officials, physicians are usually reluctant to report such instances for fear of lawsuits. The court cases that CU is aware of, however, show that delays in proper treatment have resulted in mental retardation, paralysis, and deaths from tuberculosis, spinal meningitis, and cancer.

In most of those cases, the victims were young children. The most bitter criticism of chiropractic that CU encountered, in fact, was from pediatric hospitals. Some of the reasons why were underscored in a report issued jointly in 1972 by two Canadian hospitals, the Montreal Children's Hospital and the St. Justine Hospital for Children.

The report described pamphlets distributed by chiropractors to patients in Quebec. The pamphlets claimed that chiropractors could treat epilepsy, croup, crosseye, rheumatic fever, bronchitis, pneumonia, appendicitis, leukemia, and other illnesses affecting children. Such claims, said the report, constituted "a real and direct danger" to children. "This is especially so in that many childhood illnesses are of an acute nature and require diagnosis and treatment without delay."

For example, one pamphlet then in circulation, "Chiropractic for Children," advised spinal manipulation for croup. "In actual fact," said the report of the children's hospitals, "croup is an acute infectious disease involving the voice-box area of the throat. It often requires prompt medical attention which at times may be lifesaving." Crosseye, too, should be treated at a relatively early age, or blindness may result in the affected eye, said the report.

Parents faced with a desperate situation, such as a child with leukemia, need balanced and mature advice, the report stressed. "By calling himself a 'doctor,' by taking X-Rays, by pretending to be qualified, the chiropractor creates a false image as to his ability to deal with pediatric problems. This leads directly to delay in the proper diagnosis being made and the correct therapy being started, which might affect the child for the rest of his life."

The report also decried earlier opposition of chiropractic authorities to immunization. If their position had been accepted, said the report, "then this world would now be filled with smallpox, people paralyzed [or] dead from tetanus, children choking to death from diphtheria, the uncontrolled spread of typhoid . . . and innocent children living in iron lungs because of polio."

According to a survey conducted by the ACA in August 1973, about 81 percent of its members reported that they treat children. Those chiropractors saw an average of ninety-three children annually, about 30 percent of whom were of preschool age. Respiratory ailments, allergies, and nervous-system disorders were among the most frequently treated conditions.

Each of the major chiropractic associations in the United States and Canada publishes pamphlets promoting chiropractic care for children. None of the pamphlets that CU reviewed made claims about treating infectious diseases, nor did they argue against immunization of children. But the alarm expressed in 1972 by the two Canadian children's hospitals appears to us to still be a justifiable one.

Of particular concern, in our view, is advice published in the October 1974 issue of *The ACA Journal of Chiropractic.* An article entitled "Pediatrics" recommended chiropractic treatment for children with infectious diseases, digestive disorders, respiratory illnesses, heart problems, genitourinary disorders, and other illnesses. "The infectious diseases usually respond well to chiropractic care," said the author, William A. Nelson, D.C., a charter member of the ACA. The "so-called viral diseases," he stated, "follow the same general rule," with chiropractors deciding which children to refer to physicians. "We must not lose sight of the fact that . . . our therapy is preeminent in reestablishing normal physiology where such is possible."

According to Nelson, chiropractors can also evaluate heart problems in children. "If not an acute emergency," he advised, "the easiest way may well be a short period of trial treatment." The only conditions for which he stressed medical referral among children and adolescents were acute poisoning and venereal disease.

Chiropractors use X rays to diagnose a disease process that does not exist. Even if it did, though, X rays would hardly help. Unlike bone, nerve tissue can't be seen on X rays; nor do other fine details of soft tissues stand out. Hence, what chiropractors actually look for on X rays are curvatures of the spine and departures from postural symmetry, however minor. Those are supposed to imply the presence of subluxations, which allegedly disturb nerve impulses.

But structural variations in a normal spine—as well as any shift from a perfectly straight posture just before the X ray—will also produce departures from symmetry. And those ordinary, inconsequential variations can look much the same as chiropractic "misalignments." Generally, the variations identified as misalignments by chiropractors are judged entirely normal by radiologists, who have much more extensive training in X-ray interpretation than chiropractors have. Thus, the chiropractor's X-ray diagnosis is twice removed from reality: It depends on unscientific appraisal of a nonexistent disease.

X rays can, of course, show true bone abnormalities, such as a fracture or tumor. But the 14-by-36-inch film frequently used by chiropractors for examining posture does not produce good bone detail. So, unless the chiropractor takes a smaller and more detailed view as well, abnormalities that would preclude manipulation may be missed.

Many chiropractors agree that the large film gives too little detail and too much radiation exposure. Indeed, one chiropractor quoted in the March 1975 issue of *The ACA Journal of Chiropractic* contended that "the doctor who takes such films just does it to impress the patient."

Critics of chiropractic concur and often charge that chiropractic X rays are a promotional gimmick rather than a diagnostic aid. Some chiropractic writings lend support to that allegation. A bald example appeared in the 1947 edition of *Modern X-Ray Practice and Chiropractic Spinography* by P. A. Remier, who in the mid-1960s was head of the X-ray department at Palmer College of Chiropractic. According to Remier, some of the reasons why chiropractors should X-ray "every case" were: "It promotes confidence. It creates interest among patients. It procures business. It attracts a better class of patients. It adds prestige in your community. It builds a reliable reputation."

Today, such an attitude toward radiation no longer prevails at Palmer College nor at the other two chiropractic schools CU visited. In general, the X-ray departments of those colleges appeared to teach and encourage techniques for reducing radiation exposure. But such improvements fail to get to the heart of the problem. The fact is that chiropractic X rays for "detecting subluxations" do not serve a scientifically valid purpose. In CU's opinion all such radiation is unwarranted.

Although current figures are not available, a 1971 survey by *The Journal of Clinical Chiropractic* indicated that United States and Canadian chiropractors annually took more than 10 million X rays. About 2 million of them were the 14-by-36-inch type, which irradiates the body from the skull to the thigh, including the lens of the eye, the thyroid gland, bone marrow, and the reproductive organs—four areas considered among the most susceptible to radiation damage. Evidence shows that exposure to large amounts of X ray increases the likelihood of cataracts, thyroid cancer, leukemia, and reproductive-cell damage. Public health officials are particularly concerned about the radiation dose to reproductive organs, since damage to the genetic material is a potential source of harm to future generations.

"On the average, 3 percent of people in a medical practice are X-rayed," said the Canadian children's hospitals' report. "For the chiropractor, the figure is over 90 percent." In addition, 14-by-36 full-trunk X rays account for less than one in every ten thousand hospital X rays, and the great majority of hospitals do not take full-trunk X rays at all. In contrast, about one in five chiropractic X rays is of this type.

According to a report prepared for the Canadian Association of Radiologists in May 1974, chiropractic use of full-trunk X rays is the greatest source of unnecessary gonadal radiation in Canada (especially for women, whose reproductive organs cannot be shielded from the primary X-ray beam). And chiropractic X rays were judged second only to medical and dental X rays as the leading sources of man-made radiation exposure in North America today. In CU's view, that is an extremely high risk to take for placebo medicine.

Despite the dangers of unscientific treatment, chiropractors today enjoy wider latitude in their scope of practice than any other health practitioner except the physician. By comparison, other independent health-care providers must practice within far stricter limits. A dentist doesn't treat stomach ulcers. A psychologist doesn't order medication for a heart condition. An optometrist doesn't treat epilepsy. But chiropractors may often do all three. And they are permitted to offer treatment in specialties ranging from pediatrics to psychiatry—without having scientific training in any of them. Chiropractors have won that freedom without engaging in research or demonstrating professional capability in those fields. They have won it by one method alone: political action.

For years, grass roots politics has been the lifeblood of chiropractic. By marshaling the support of chiropractic patients, the profession has often achieved an effective political voice in legislation affecting its licensure and services. And that voice has been its protection against science. Opponents of chiropractic come to legislative hearings armed with information, scientific studies, and official statements from national organizations. Chiropractors come armed with votes.

The inclusion of chiropractic services under Medicare, after a seven-year campaign by chiropractors and their supporters, provides a classic example. Against the combined opposition of the AMA, the U.S. Department of Health, Education, and Welfare, the National Council of Senior Citizens, and numerous other groups, the chiropractic lobby emphasized one primary weapon: the mailbox. Congressional aides were reportedly astonished over the sacks of pro-chiropractic mail that didn't seem to diminish. It got the message across.

In its eighty-five-year war with science, chiropractic has won the major battles. Recently, chiropractors have gained even more ground in skirmishes against organized medicine by taking the AMA to court. In several states, including Illinois, New Jersey, New York, and Pennsylvania, chiropractors have kept the AMA busy defending lawsuits holding it in restraint of trade. Such tactics undoubtedly helped chiropractic win its latest victory—a breach in the AMA's long-standing ban on chiropractic as "an unscientific cult" to be shunned by physicians. At the AMA's annual meeting in Chicago in July 1979 members of the House of Delegates voted, in effect, to let individual physicians decide whether or not to refer patients to chiropractors or accept chiropractic referrals. At the same time, the AMA reaffirmed its position that chiropractic should play no part in the diagnosis and treatment of certain diseases, among them cancer, diabetes, heart disease, and hypertension.

Ultimately, chiropractors seek to gain inclusion under any future national health insurance program. In the past, the public's freedom to choose among health practitioners has been honored in legislation affecting chiropractors. CU believes that principle will be sustained if a national health insurance bill emerges. Before such services are included, however, we think that public safety demands a searching review and thorough reform of chiropractic practices by appropriate state and federal agencies.

Recommendations

Overall, Consumers Union believes that chiropractic is a significant hazard to many patients. Current licensing laws, in our opinion, lend an aura of legitimacy to unscientific practices and serve to protect the chiropractor rather than the public. In effect, those laws allow persons with limited qualifications to practice medicine under another name.

We believe the public health would be better served if state and federal governments used their licensing authority and their power of the purse to restrict the chiropractor's scope of practice more effectively. Specifically, we think that licensing laws and federal health insurance programs should limit chiropractic treatment to appropriate musculoskeletal complaints and ban *all* chiropractic use of X rays and drugs, including nutritional supplements, for the purported treatment of disease. Above all, we would urge that chiropractors be prohibited from treating children; children do not have the freedom to reject an unscientific therapy that their parents may mistakenly turn to for help in a crisis.

If you've been considering a chiropractor for the first time, we think it would be safer for you to reconsider. Even if you are dissatisfied with your physician's treatment of a back problem, you can ask for a consultation with another physician, such as an orthopedist or physiatrist (a specialist in physical medicine). Then, if manipulative treatment were indicated, it could be performed by that specialist or by a physical therapist.

Despite this recommendation, we recognize that some people will still decide to use the services of a chiropractor. For those who do, and who wish to avoid some of the dubious practices that occur, we think some advice given to CU by chiropractic officials themselves may be helpful.

☐Avoid any practitioner who makes claims about cures,

either orally or in advertising. Anyone who implies or promises guaranteed results from treatment should be held suspect.

☐Beware of chiropractors who ask you to sign a contract for services. A written agreement is not customary practice.

☐Reject anyone advertising free X rays. Radiation should not be used as a lure.

☐Ask whether the chiropractor refers patients to other health professionals. If the answer is "No"—or if the chiropractor disparages other professions or accepted treatment—walk out.

☐Don't make advance payments. Most chiropractors have a flat office fee and don't offer "discounts" for prepayment. Nor is it accepted practice to charge extra for "units of treatment," such as manipulation, heat therapy, and the like. That should be included in the office fee.

☐Don't be pressured by scare tactics, such as threats of "irreversible damage" if treatment isn't begun promptly. And watch out for those who encourage "intensive treatment" because anything less would be a "patch-up job." The intensive treatment is more likely to apply to your bank account.

CU would add one more precaution: See a physician as well and find out what he or she has to say about the problem.

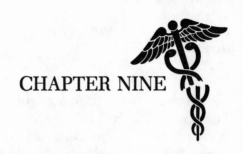

CHAPTER NINE

Mail-Order
Health Frauds

*Step right up, folks, and welcome to the **Mail-Order
Health Carnival!** It's sponsored by some of America's
leading **Newspapers** and **Magazines**. Better yet, folks,
you don't even have to stand up and be counted. Now,
in the privacy of your own home, or in the comfort of
your sickbed, while thumbing through your favorite
magazines and newspapers, you can select dozens of
widely self-acclaimed nostrums to accommodate your
every **Health** and **Sex** fantasy!*

*You say your face bags, your belly sags, your hair
lags? Just whip out your checkbook, and you can send
away for the most **Amazing** wrinkle removers, the most
Ingenious girdles, the most POTENT baldness cures,
and the most **Astounding** bust developers!*

*You say you live in mortal terror of forty (count 'em,
40) dread diseases? Well, cheer up, folks, because the
best is yet to come. **For a Limited Time Only,** you can
place your order for the most **Fabulously** outrageous
medical advice available today. You'll learn about a*

Health Quackery

Secret Cure *for arthritis, diabetes, and, yes, even heart disease!!!*
This way, ladies and gentlemen, right this way!

Although the horse-drawn wagons are gone, the health pitchman's carnival is still thriving. And today's cast numbers in the thousands. Many have just walk-on roles—the fly-by-nighters who place an ad, open a post office box, wait until the checks roll in, and then vanish before the authorities can catch up with them. The real stars of the show, though, are certain big mail-order houses that peddle dozens of worthless products.

It may come as no surprise that the age-old carnival of quackery is still barnstorming its way through the pockets of the gullible and the desperate. But it's a deep frustration to those charged with protecting the public to find that much of the health-and-sex carnival atmosphere exudes from the pages of reputable magazines and newspapers.

In mid-1977 and early 1978, eighteen national magazines, including *Sports Illustrated* and *Esquire,* carried a full-page ad for a plastic belt: "The most astounding Waistline Reducer of all time! *Astro-Trimmer* . . . Guaranteed to reduce your waistline 2 to 4 inches in just 3 days-or-less. . . ."

Headlines of a full-page ad that ran in October 1978 in twelve big-city papers, including *The Washington Post* and *The Los Angeles Times,* declared: "BURNS AWAY MORE FAT EACH 24 HOURS THAN IF YOU RAN 14 MILES A DAY! Incredible Crash-Loss Breakthrough Reported in Leading American Magazines! Works So Fast You Can Actually Measure the Difference In Your Waistline In Just 24 to 48 Hours! . . . The name of this wondrous amino formula is THERA-SLIM-100. . . ." An essentially similar advertisement appeared in *TV Guide, Woman's Day,* and other major magazines.

A full-page ad in the October 1978 issue of *Cosmopolitan* told readers about the following prospect: "Your bust will grow right before your eyes . . . and grow . . . and grow . . . and grow with the sensational *MARK EDEN MARK II Bust Developer with IVR.* . . . Already a rumble is starting from west to east about this startling innovation . . . about the bust developer everybody said could never be perfected. . . . *You must see a visible improvement on your bust . . . the very first time you use the* Mark Eden Mark II with IVR *and you must add up to 3 or more inches on your bust the very first week or your money back."* Slightly different ads for an earlier model *Mark Eden* appeared in nineteen other national magazines, among them *Mademoiselle, Photoplay,* and *Redbook.*

In view of the cost of such advertising—a full-page, black-and-white ad in *Cosmopolitan* ran about $13,000 —the promoters must place the ads with high hopes of finding marks. Evidently, their hopes are realized. *Mark Eden* boasted in a May 1978 ad that it had sold 4 million bust developers at $9.95 each. That adds up to something like $40 million—not bad for a product made essentially of two pieces of plastic held together by a spring.

Probably the most extensive study of mail-order health advertising was done in the summer of 1977 by the quackery committee of the Pennsylvania Medical

Health Quackery

Society. The committee screened five hundred nationally circulated magazines and found that about a quarter of them carried ads for mail-order health products. Altogether, about one hundred fifty such products were offered by fifty promoters. The products included weight reducers, bust developers, blemish removers, hair-loss remedies, longevity formulas, aphrodisiacs, sexual pleasure enhancers, penis extenders, and impotency aids. Despite their various alleged purposes, almost all those products had one thing in common: The physicians judged their ads to be misleading.

Similarly, the three products whose ads we quoted on pages 202–203 also share a common bond: A U.S. Food and Drug Administration physician working with the U.S. Postal Service officially advised the Postal Service that the advertisements for all three products were deceptive and misleading.

The Postal Service has responsibility for protecting the public from deceptions and frauds involving use of the mails. Five inspectors in the agency's Special Investigation Division concentrate on cases involving mail-order health schemes. There are more than enough cases to keep them busy. The agency's law department brings about one hundred fifty actions each year, but the sheer number of health promotions allows many health schemes to go uncurbed. According to Postal Service estimates, mail-order health fraud costs Americans at least $150 million a year.

Most of the legal actions taken are settled through compromise agreement. The promoter agrees to change or halt the advertising, and the Postal Service withdraws its complaint. When no compromise can be reached, the agency can issue a "stop order," causing all mail for the product to be returned to senders.

Postal officials say that there are three common misconceptions about mail-order health products: First, that the Postal Service licenses mail-order advertisers; second, that health advice published in magazines and books must be legitimate; and, third, that ads appearing in a reputable magazine or newspaper must be valid. None of these assumptions is true, say postal officials. The mistaken belief about ads appearing in reputable publications is the most galling of all to those trying to protect the public from fraudulent products.

Many newspapers that pride themselves on the accuracy and reliability of their news coverage print mail-order health ads without checking even the most outrageous claims. In January 1978, for example, some 2 million copies of a four-page brochure were accepted for insertion into the various editions of eighteen city newspapers from coast to coast.* The brochure promoted a handbook, "Modern Solution to Age Old Physical Problems," published by the Midwest Health Research Laboratory. The handbook, it was claimed, "contained a solution or prevention for as many as forty (40) different diseases and illnesses," including arthritis, diabetes, and hardening of the arteries. More than one thousand readers surrendered to the inviting logic of the promotion: "Our special introductory offer of $9.95

Tampa Tribune, St. Paul Dispatch, Seattle Post-Intelligencer, Dallas Times Herald, Houston Chronicle, Houston Post, Oakland Tribune, Erie Times-News, Raleigh News & Observer, Bogalusa (La.) News, Spartanburg (S.C.) Herald-Journal, San Antonio Express-News, Atlantic City Press, Port Huron (Mich.) Times Herald, Gadsden (Ala.) Times, New Ulm (Minn.) Journal, Council Bluffs (Iowa) Nonpareil, and Pasadena Star-News.

can save you unnecessary visits to the doctor, the hospital, and save you money."

Those who mailed money received a twenty-five-page booklet revealing the secret cure-all and end-all of disease—"colonic irrigation," otherwise known as an enema, preferably "two to three times a week." Coupons were available for those desiring "personal Home Treatment Kits" at $29.95 apiece.

Eventually, complaints began arriving at Postal Service offices. None of the people who ordered the handbook got their money back, but the Postal Service was in time to stop orders for the kits. A doctor who testified at a Postal Service hearing underlined the gravity of the fraud; he said that enemas could be extremely dangerous in certain illnesses, such as colitis and appendicitis. The promoter behind Midwest Health, one Shane G. Brannson III, alias Robert B. Goode, was indicted by a Kansas City, Missouri, grand jury on eighteen criminal counts, including two counts of mail fraud. In a plea-bargain arrangement, Brannson pleaded guilty to two counts and was sentenced to three years in prison, to be followed by four years' probation. Among the complaints received by the Postal Service were several from newspapers that hadn't been paid for running the Midwest Health ads.

Readers rooked by this scheme had trust in their local paper and believed that a product it advertised would be legitimate. But many newspapers and magazines that carry mail-order health ads require from the advertiser nothing more than payment for the space. As the enema promotion shows, even that requirement is sometimes overlooked.

Mail-Order Health Frauds

A publication's failure to screen its health ads can cost more than money. In 1977 *Mothering Magazine* published an ad for "She-Link Herbal Pill No. 9, the amazing Herbal Pill for long-term birth control." Those ordering She-Link received eight pills with instructions to take them all at one time to prevent conception for six months. At the request of the Postal Service, the Food and Drug Administration investigated and later ruled that the pill was a "spurious contraceptive which poses a serious health hazard to women." Corroborating the FDA findings was evidence that eighty-seven women—two of them on the *Mothering Magazine* staff—had become pregnant after taking the pills. The promoter of the deceptive contraceptive, Gee Singh Tong, was sentenced to three years in prison for mail fraud.

Yet many deceptive advertisers manage to sidestep the Postal Service. Some simply pocket their earnings and disappear when they're discovered. They may surface again after changing their address, the ownership of their company, or the name of their product. Others may consent to stop a particular promotion and then create another gimmick with slightly different claims. The Postal Service is obliged to treat each variation of the original deception as a new violation—a costly and time-consuming process. Further, imprisonment or a fine can result only from a successful criminal action. And criminal actions are even more costly and difficult. The government must not only prove that deceptions were intentional but also must usually find people willing to testify against a particular mail-order product. Few fraud victims are eager to stand up in open court and admit to having been gulled. For three years, the

Health Quackery

Postal Service was anxious to press charges against a company that was successfully marketing a penis extender. But during that time it received only one complaint—for nondelivery of the product.

Some products sold through direct mail can be dangerous if put to use by an unwary consumer. Agencies such as the Postal Service often do not find out that these schemes exist. One product the Postal Service did learn about was the "Algamar" cancer cure, a home treatment kit costing $697. The kit consisted of two vials of liquid "kelp vitamin complex," a bottle of brown vitamin pills, and several hypodermic syringes. The kit was purported to cure not only cancer, but also cardiovascular disorders, epilepsy, emphysema, and hepatitis.

Analysis of the vials showed they contained large quantities of two bacteria that can cause serious illness or death. The Postal Service was able to track down several customers, some of whom had already died from cancer. The "inventor" of the kit, Thomas C. Johnstone, was characterized by prosecutors as having taken "incredible liberties with other people's lives." Indicted for mail fraud, Johnstone was sentenced in U.S. District Court in January 1978 to three years' probation, fined $1,000, and ordered to devote one hundred hours to community work.

A few years ago, seven federal agencies commissioned a study of the health practices and opinions of the American people. The survey, published in 1972, came to this conclusion: "Substantial numbers of people believe that advertisers, in the health field as elsewhere, are watched and regulated closely enough so that serious distortions are unlikely and outright fabrications are nearly impossible. There is a feeling that 'they wouldn't dare' make up 'evidence' to support a claim, or falsify testimonials, for example, because 'they would be caught.' " But many *do* dare, and many *don't* get caught. So, considering the limits of government regulation, the basic question of responsibility remains.

Just who *is* responsible for ensuring the integrity of ads appearing in newspapers and magazines? The logical candidates would appear to be the advertiser, the publisher, or both. Quite predictably, neither party wants the honor. *Advertising Age,* the influential marketing trade publication, has long urged newspapers and magazines to clean up deceptive advertisements in their pages. A 1975 *Advertising Age* editorial combined the exhortation with a warning: "Most Americans believe owners of reputable media make at least some effort to check their advertisers, and it is this consumer credibility that media often stress to advertisers who want to be seen in good company. . . . However painful the alternative, media owners cannot escape the fact that their failure to screen out dubious ads plays into the hands of those who are telling the Federal Trade Commission and other agencies that media must be held accountable for injury incurred by readers or viewers who respond to those ads."

But publishers apparently aren't interested in accepting such a role. According to a representative of the American Newspaper Publishers Association, the responsibility for an ad lies squarely on the advertiser. Although newspapers have no obligation to do so, "most try to see that an ad is legitimate," according to

Health Quackery

Donald R. McVay, senior vice president of the publishers' association. Consumers Union asked McVay if his trade organization had any advertising code to guide its members. "You'll never get a code or regulation out of us," he said. "It's not a function of our organization. It's entirely up to the individual publisher." McVay mailed us a 1974 survey, conducted by the publishers' group, on "how newspapers protect integrity of advertising." A major conclusion from the survey: "More than 90 percent of daily newspapers have some form of code or set of standards which they follow in determining advertising acceptability."

What sort of code or standards do individual publishers set for themselves? Many publications claim that they screen ads carefully, but CU found reason to be skeptical about that. Bob Martin, customer relations manager for *The Washington Post*, told us that the *Post* has an advertising acceptance committee that "screens copy that comes in for all mail-order advertising." He said the committee "checks for blatant, outrageous claims." Yet the *Post* and eleven other prominent publications carried full-page ads for *Thera-Slim-100*, the "diet aid" that supposedly "burns away more fat each 24 hours than if you ran 14 miles a day."

Jack Kerrigan, the *Post*'s general advertising manager, said, "We generally check out products like diet fads and turn a lot of them down." Yet the *Post* ran the *Thera-Slim-100* ads at least four times in the summer and fall of 1978, despite the fact that its promoter, American Consumer Inc., has been the target of numerous state and federal actions. Kerrigan said the *Post* was aware of actions taken against American Consumer, and if the company had been found guilty of any charges, the *Post* would stop accepting its ads.

For the record, in the spring of 1977 American Consumer paid a total of $94,000 in fines, civil penalties, and court costs to the states of Pennsylvania and California because of false and misleading advertising and other offenses. From February 1975 through October 1978 the Postal Service brought fourteen actions against American Consumer. Nine were settled by compromise; in five others, mail-stop orders were issued after an administrative law judge ruled the company had violated postal statutes. Between November 1978 and July 1979 twelve additional cases were filed, all against American Consumer; of these, eight have already resulted in consent agreements, and mail-stop orders were issued in two other cases.

In June 1977 the U.S. Justice Department, acting on behalf of the FDA, seized three American Consumer health products for false and misleading labeling. The Justice Department has asked a Federal District Court in Pennsylvania to force American Consumer in the future to submit its proposed labeling for any food, cosmetic, or medical device to the FDA with supporting medical documentation. The unusual request was made, according to a Justice Department attorney, because the company continues to sell mislabeled products despite previous actions against it. As part of the same action, the Justice Department seized six American Consumer products—including *Thera-Slim-100*—with a total retail value of $670,000. The FDA alleged that the labels on these products were false and misleading.

Health Quackery

Mail-order houses like American Consumer depend largely on newspapers and magazines to carry their advertising messages. And the publications certainly cooperate. In October 1978 we sampled twenty-five different newspapers. Twelve carried full-page ads for *Thera-Slim-100* and eight more carried ads for other American Consumer products. Thanks to that kind of exposure, American Consumer has been doing very well. It reportedly takes in more than $30 million a year.

According to Stephen Barrett, M.D., who headed the Pennsylvania Medical Society's mail-order health investigation, *Cosmopolitan* apparently derives more income from questionable health ads than any other magazine. The *Cosmopolitan* mail-order manager, Robert Nesbit, told CU that the magazine makes an effort to screen the ads it prints. "We screen for good taste and for anything we feel will be fraudulent or a rip-off," he said. Yet *Cosmopolitan*'s October 1978 issue alone ran ads for eleven products that have prompted investigations or actions by the Postal Service.

Nesbit has little regard for the Postal Service, terming it a "kangaroo court." According to Nesbit, his magazine doesn't have the resources to screen all its ads. It presumably doesn't need to, because it "insists" that all the mail-order products advertised in it carry a money-back guarantee with no time restriction for returning the product for a refund. "If you order something through the pages of *Cosmopolitan,* you can't lose," said Nesbit. The guarantee for the *Mark Eden Bust Developer* we ordered from an ad in *Cosmopolitan* stipulates: "All returns must be postmarked not later

than 14 days from the patron's receipt of her course."
A thirty-day limit applies to *NutraNail,* a *Cosmopolitan*-advertised nail grower. For *Biotin Solution Hair Restoration Gel,* another product with a full page in the magazine, there's no guarantee at all.

Do money-back guarantees reduce an ad's deception? A Federal Trade Commission official told us that the FTC is considering action against, among other things, some mail-order health products whose ads include money-back guarantees. Such guarantees are themselves deceptive, the FTC official points out, because they suggest that the product is effective.

We asked Nesbit about three bust developers, advertised in the October 1978 *Cosmopolitan,* that were under investigation by the Postal Service. Nesbit said it was a funny thing about bust developers: They don't work for all women, but only for "certain kinds"—tall, thin women. The statement is interesting not for what it says about bust developers (medical testimony in several court cases emphasizes that bust developers are ineffective for *all* women), but for what it says about *Cosmopolitan*'s self-policing. Assuming Nesbit believes that bust developers work only for tall, thin women, he must be aware that the ads in *Cosmopolitan,* which suggest that these products can help *any* woman, are at least a little off base.

Newspapers and magazines have the First Amendment right of freedom of speech. They cannot and should not be told what to print or not print. But this freedom combined with commercially motivated lack of concern about mail-order health advertising leaves many consumers deceived and defrauded. It makes little sense to ask mail-order advertisers—whose livelihood may depend on deception—to police their own ads. Improvement in this area can only come with self-regulation on the part of the publishers.

Some officials of the American Newspaper Publishers Association proposed in November 1978 that newspapers and magazines establish central clearinghouses to help members spot potentially fraudulent ads. Such clearinghouses could draw up ad "profiles," which would alert advertising departments to possible problems. Conceivably, such profiles could rely in part on the extensive medical testimony from Postal Service hearings and court cases. In addition, clearinghouses could check the Postal Service's quarterly enforcement reports to find out which products may be violating the law.

Many publishers contend that screening ads is too time-consuming and difficult. If that's the case, we urge that they print disclaimers next to their ads, indicating that they can't vouch for the claims made in their pages. That way consumers might not be duped into buying worthless products merely because they respect the publication printing the ad.

Congress could also help by giving the Postal Service the authority to levy civil penalties. Fines that match profits would help eliminate the financial incentive to engage in deceptive practices. At present, mail-order con artists can be fined only as a result of criminal prosecution. Civil penalties would be less cumbersome and expensive than criminal prosecution and could result in more timely action against all mail frauds, not just the health frauds.

Even with that added weapon, the Postal Service could only partly control mail-order health deceptions. And so far, many newspapers and magazines are not willing to screen the ads they publish. So consumers must rely on their own judgment to guard against mail-order health fraud.

The best rule-of-thumb is this: If something sounds too good to be true, it probably is. CU's medical consultants offer the following guidelines to help consumers who may be tempted by mail-order health advertising.

□Bust developers. The only muscles in the female breast are in the nipple, so there's not much to "develop." Exercise may enlarge the back muscles and, to a lesser extent, the pectoral muscles underlying the breasts, producing a slightly increased chest measurement. But growth of the breasts themselves is influenced only by hormones—released during puberty and pregnancy—and by general weight gain. Mark Eden, a major producer of bust developers, promised to send us "medical documentation" that its product works. We're still waiting.

□Penis extenders. Like the breast, the penis contains no muscles to be developed by vacuum pumps or whatever.

□Wrinkle removers. No cream or liquid that's safe to put on the skin can do more than temporarily increase the water content of the skin, and then only to the point of masking the most superficial of wrinkles. "Anti-aging" pills containing RNA, DNA, or other chemicals have no beneficial effect at all. Only plastic surgery can remove wrinkles for any length of time.

□Baldness remedies. Male pattern baldness, the most

common type of baldness, is hereditary. Medical science knows of no pill or cream that can arrest that genetically determined condition. In some instances, loss of hair may also be symptomatic of various emotional and physical disorders.

☐Aphrodisiacs. Most pills and powders with aphrodisiacal pretensions contain "Spanish fly," a legendary ingredient celebrated for its purported effect on women. Today's "Spanish fly" consists mainly of red pepper. It causes nothing more than mild irritation of the urethra. The ginseng root, long used as an Oriental cure-all, has recently acquired a reputation in this country for improving sexual prowess. The FDA has unearthed no evidence to support the root's reputation.

☐Diet pills, protein supplements, reducing devices. There is no proof that such gimmicks are effective for weight loss. Most nonprescription diet pills contain either phenylpropanolamine or methylcellulose. Some evidence indicates phenylpropanolamine can act as an appetite suppressant, but only for short periods. Methylcellulose is a "bulking agent," which supposedly expands in the stomach to relieve hunger pangs. There's no evidence that it works. Weight-loss powders are usually accompanied by instructions bidding users to follow a rigid low-calorie diet as well. The diet might very well promote a weight loss, but the protein products contribute nothing. Clinical studies by the FDA have shown that "body wraps"—devices wrapped around parts of the body for selective weight loss—are useless. Some can be harmful.

☐Megavitamins. Everyone recognizes that adequate amounts of vitamins are necessary for *good* health. But no one has ever shown that extra large or "megavitamin" doses produce *better* health. Depending on the vitamin, amounts beyond the National Academy of Sciences/National Research Council's Recommended Daily Allowances can be dangerous or just a waste of money. Too much of the fat-soluble vitamins A and D can build up in the body to dangerous levels. Doses of water-soluble vitamins that exceed what the body can use are simply excreted in the urine.

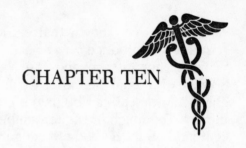

CHAPTER TEN

Nutrition as Therapy

"Our frying-pans and gridirons slay more than the sword," exclaimed John Adams during the American Revolution. He was lamenting the drab diet and food shortages of the time, especially in the armies. Today some critics of the American diet view it with similar distress. Their complaint is not with a paucity of foods, however, but a paucity of nutrients. Americans, they say, are not getting enough of the vital substances they need to prevent disease and experience robust good health.

Part of the criticism, Consumers Union believes, may be true for some people: Economic hardship, lack of nutrition education, and heavy promotion of highly processed or "junk" foods by industry may sometimes lead to inadequate diets, especially among the poor, the very young, and the elderly. But most Americans are not undernourished. They obtain enough—and often far more than enough—of the nutrients they need.

Several well-defined disorders arise from nutritional

deficiencies, but that fact has been distorted into the notion that *many* diseases result from inadequate nutrition—and can be prevented or cured by taking large doses of vitamins and other food supplements, or by following odd dietary regimens. Not surprisingly, a thriving enterprise in nutritional "therapies" has developed.

Thus, Americans are variously urged to banish certain staple foods or favor others. They are told to shun meat, or white bread, or tomatoes, or whatever, and to fill up on garlic, fiber, alfalfa tablets, or herbs. They are advised to swallow enormous quantities of calcium, vitamin C, vitamin E, zinc, and a host of other food supplements. Whatever the menu advocated, it is invariably supposed to prevent human ills or to restore the body to bristling vitality.

According to this view, food no longer serves merely as nourishment or as a source of pleasure. It is the sovereign remedy for disease. Depending on the particular advocate, various foods and food supplements will purportedly clean out the arteries, cure arthritis, stop hair from thinning, spark sex life, prevent cancer, sharpen vision, fight depression, shore up the bones, and restore adolescent vigor.

Such claims help support a multibillion-dollar business in so-called health foods, dietary supplements, and nutrition publications.

The idea that food can serve as more than just nourishment is as old as human history. A belief in the mystical healing power of garlic, for instance, dates back to ancient Egypt and has been periodically exhumed since the days of the Greeks. At various times, maple sugar, asparagus, coffee, and pineapple were viewed as therapeutic panaceas. Potatoes, on the other hand, were shunned as poisonous when Sir Walter Raleigh brought them from America to Europe, as were turnips, beets, and tomatoes.

In the absence of scientific knowledge, folklore and superstition often served as a guide to the healing or harmful properties ascribed to food. Occasionally, a food remedy was on target, as when surgeon's mate James Lind demonstrated in 1747 that lemon juice could be used to prevent or treat scurvy among British sailors. More often, however, such remedies offered no real benefits. Indeed, the science of nutrition is essentially a child of the twentieth century.

Around the turn of the century, research in the Far East and England suggested that some diseases might arise from a lack of certain nutrients in the diet. In 1911, Casimir Funk, a Polish chemist working in London, coined the word "vitamine" to describe such substances. E. V. McCollum, a biochemist at the University of Wisconsin, identified the first vitamin—vitamin A— in 1913. Researchers throughout the world discovered other vitamins, and the knowledge ultimately led to a sharp reduction in the incidence of vitamin deficiency diseases, such as beriberi, rickets, and pellagra.

The discovery of vitamins captured the public's imagination and sparked wide interest in nutrition. But, observed James Harvey Young, Ph.D., professor of history at Emory University and a leading authority on health quackery, the new revelations could easily be twisted and distorted to provoke alarm. "Even while eating enough of what you usually ate, you might get sick. To stay healthy some mysterious extras might be needed. You couldn't see them and you couldn't taste them, but without them you might acquire horrendous symptoms or else just wither away."

During the 1920s, reported Young, "the word vitamin appeared with increasing frequency in food advertising, even for chocolate bars." And multivitamin "cures" for high blood pressure, kidney disease, and other disorders began receiving widespread promotion.

By the 1940s, scientists had identified more than forty nutrients, including thirteen vitamins and various trace elements, thus multiplying the candidates for promotion. The wartime food-enrichment program further publicized vitamins. And a vigorous campaign by the U.S. Food and Drug Administration against traditional forms of medical quackery drove hard-pressed promoters into the more respectable "nutrition" business.

Events of the 1960s increased the nation's receptivity to food faddism, especially among the young. The Vietnam War, assassinations, and political turmoil brought disillusion with government, business, and other institutions. Establishment science, which had spawned the nuclear bomb, napalm, and environment-threatening chemicals, was held equally suspect. One outcome was a back-to-nature movement, which the growing health food industry and some major food marketers were quick to exploit.

Ultimately, however, it was Congress itself that handed food-fad promoters their most stunning victory. In 1976 a bill championed by Senator William

Proxmire of Wisconsin effectively scuttled the FDA's authority to regulate the marketing of vitamins and other food supplements. In an intensive lobbying effort, the health food industry had generated some 2 million letters to Congress in support of the legislation, and Congress responded. Among its provisions, the bill prohibited the FDA from requiring that dietary supplements contain nutritionally essential vitamins and minerals or that the products exclude "useless ingredients with no nutritional value." The bill was "a charlatan's dream," said Alexander M. Schmidt, FDA commissioner at the time. "Somebody could bottle sawdust and sell it as a food supplement."

In theory, the public still has a measure of protection against a sawdust marketer: It would be illegal for the marketer to make false health claims in the labeling or advertising of the product. In practice, however, that safeguard is often illusory, because another and more fundamental law works to the promoter's advantage.

Constitutional protection of freedom of speech and the press covers the publication of nonsense about nutrition as well as scientific discussions of it. Editorial material may freely propound false, misleading, or deceptive health information, as long as there's no link to the promotion of a specific product (as in an advertisement). Books and magazine articles can claim miraculous cures for various wonder diets without good evidence, and self-ordained "nutrition experts" can do the same on radio and television.

Indirectly, marketers of dietary supplements can derive a promotional advantage from the constitutional protection afforded the press. While prohibited by law from making unproved health claims in their ads, they can place those ads in publications that specialize in articles attributing great health benefits to the very products advertised. The claims made in the editorial text may then seem to embrace the advertisers' wares.

Each month, for example, *Prevention* magazine prints several articles extolling the virtues of various vitamins, minerals, and health food fads, such as bone meal, amaranth, garlic, and alfalfa. The articles often fail to distinguish between nutritional fact and fiction. Claims judged by CU's medical consultants as being unproved or discredited (vitamin E is a treatment for heart disease, vitamin C prevents cancer) are often given credence or even enthusiastic support in *Prevention.*

Advertising space in *Prevention* is not cheap. As of October 1979, the general advertising rate was $12,355 for a black-and-white page, $21,715 for a color page, and $28,225 for the back cover. Despite the high costs, several 1979 issues of the magazine have carried each month at least one hundred pages of ads (including inserts), nearly all of which were devoted to food supplements, health food nostrums, and related products.

Food-fad promoters, in short, have a decided edge over the unwary consumer. Unregulated in any practical way, they have broad latitude in exploiting a nutrition-conscious marketplace. Another crucial factor in the successful promotion of food nostrums, however, is the state of nutrition knowledge itself.

Surveys of the public consistently disclose widespread misinformation, ignorance, or confusion about nutrition. But the public is not alone in its confusion.

Health Quackery

Nutrition scientists themselves have only a limited understanding of the role that diet may play in preventing or alleviating disease. While much is already known about what nutrients people need for good nourishment, scientific knowledge of the effects that specific diets may have on health is still incomplete.

The role of diet in cancer is a typical example. Scientists generally agree that dietary patterns do influence the incidence of certain types of cancer. The question is how. As studies among Seventh-Day Adventists have indicated, the answers can be elusive. Seventh-Day Adventists are a popular group for scientific study because their lifestyle differs sharply from that of most other Americans. By church proscription, almost all Adventists abstain from alcohol and tobacco. About half are also vegetarians, most of whom eat eggs and dairy foods but no meat, poultry, or fish of any kind. About 2 percent are strict vegetarians, who use no animal products at all.

A long-term study of Adventists conducted by the Loma Linda University School of Medicine in California found that the group experienced a much lower incidence of cancer than the United States population as a whole. Prevalence rates of cancers that are strongly associated with smoking or alcohol were extremely low. Lung cancer, for example, was only 20 percent of the national rate. The rates of some cancers believed to be associated with diet were also lower than the national rate, though not to the same degree. The rate of colon cancer, for example, was 72 percent of that for the general population.

Colon cancer is of special interest because some studies suggest that it is associated with diets low in fiber (the "roughage" in fruit, vegetables, and cereals) and high in meat and other animal products. Because of their large percentage of vegetarians, Adventists as a group consume, on average, more fiber and less meat than people in the general population. Consequently, their lower rate of colon cancer might seem to bear out the theory that meat and fiber intake are associated with the disease.

A closer look, however, reveals why nutrition scientists are often loath to jump to conclusions. When the vegetarian Adventists were compared with the non-vegetarians, there was no difference in colon cancer rates between the two groups. The Adventists were also compared with the Mormons, another religious group that proscribes alcohol and tobacco but whose diet includes meat and is not significantly different from that of the general population. The Mormons' rate of colon cancer was found to be just as low as that of the Adventists.

Such ambiguities in nutrition lead many scientists to question any blanket dietary recommendations not based on conclusive scientific proof. Evidence is not commonly judged conclusive until several well-controlled, independent studies show consistent results. Weight-reducing diets for obese diabetics, for example, will consistently lessen or even eliminate the need for medication, just as sodium-restricted diets will consistently aid in the treatment of congestive heart failure. The evidence in both instances is clear-cut and conclusive.

No such proof exists for many publicized notions linking diet to certain diseases. Despite numerous books offering dietary panaceas for arthritis, there is no scientific evidence that such measures either prevent or cure the disease. Nor is there any substantiated scientific basis for claims that sugar causes diabetes or that various dietary supplements or unusual food combinations can reduce the risk of heart attack, cancer, or numerous other diseases.

"Scientific evidence" cited by food-fad promoters often tends to be outdated or discredited reports or preliminary results that are still unconfirmed. Claims that vitamin E benefits heart patients, for example, are based on reports publicized a generation ago (see Chapter Five) and subsequently discredited.

Sometimes food-fad promoters will cite legitimate evidence but exaggerate or misinterpret it for their purpose. If a study finds little heart disease among aborigines eating high-fiber foods, it will be touted as a compelling reason for people to rush out and stock up on bran tablets or apple pectose wafers. Fiber is currently presented as one of the miracle cures for a host of human ills. Actually, its value is established only for constipation and for diverticular disease, an ailment of the bowel.

Vitamins are deservedly popular among retailers. According to a November 1978 report in *Drug Topics,* a trade journal for pharmacists, the markup on vitamin products averaged about 43 percent in drugstores; in health food outlets the average markup was even higher. Vitamins and other food supplements ring up an estimated $1.2 billion in sales annually, reported *Drug Topics.* "For the small amount of space it requires, nothing equals the vitamin section for fast turnover . . . and large profits."

Do the benefits of vitamin supplements accrue to the user as well as the seller, though? No one disputes the role of vitamins in maintaining normal health. But the amounts needed are relatively modest and can generally be obtained from a balanced diet of foods and minimal exposure to sunshine.

Magazines like *Prevention* and *The Body Forum,* however, frequently proclaim that vitamins in large doses ("megavitamins") will prevent real or imagined ills that an ordinary diet cannot handle. The scientific literature tells another story. Despite numerous claims for the wonders of large vitamin doses, especially of vitamins C and E, the evidence for such results is meager indeed. Over the years, the benefits claimed have consistently failed to materialize under close scientific scrutiny.

In well-controlled studies, megadoses of vitamin C failed to prevent or cure colds as advertised. Claims that it could help cancer patients have now been tested and found wanting. In a clinical trail at the Mayo Clinic in Rochester, Minnesota, reported in 1979, high-dose vitamin C failed to support assertions that it could prolong or improve the lives of terminal cancer patients. "We cannot now identify any therapeutic benefit of such a course," said Edward T. Creagan, M.D. of the clinic.

Trials of vitamin E have been no less disappointing. High doses of the vitamin have failed to show benefit in so many instances that it is still known as "a vitamin in search of a disease." A modest requirement for vitamin E—readily available from many vegetables and vegetable oils, margarine, cereals, fish, and numerous other sources in an ordinary diet—has been established by the National Academy of Sciences. But the therapeutic efficacy of the vitamin has been proved conclusively in only one illness, a rare type of anemia in premature infants. Meanwhile, research on vitamin E has not revealed it to be of any value in the treatment of miscarriages, sterility, menopausal disturbances, muscular dystrophies, cystic fibrosis, blood disorders, leg ulcers, diabetes, and a variety of heart and vascular diseases.

Claims that schizophrenia and minimal brain dysfunction could be successfully treated with large doses of vitamins have met a similar fate. Several carefully controlled trials have evaluated megavitamin therapy in schizophrenia and found no benefit. Indeed, the studies suggested possible adverse effects, such as longer periods in the hospital, increased need for other drugs, and poorer post-hospital adjustment. In general, the treatment was judged to be inferior to a placebo (dummy medication).

A trial of megavitamins among children with minimal brain dysfunction, reported in 1978, produced no significant differences between the vitamin group and a control group receiving placebos. Only two children responded so well that further medication was considered unnecessary; both were in the placebo group. To date, none of the numerous claims touting significant therapeutic benefits from megavitamins has been confirmed by well-controlled clinical studies.

Minerals have been another "miracle" commodity

for food-fad promoters. Zinc may be only a poor relation of gold in the mineral world, but in the health food market it has financial clout. Along with calcium, another mineral, it has joined the current rank of favorites among food-supplement marketers.

Because of their varied roles in the body, both minerals are ideal candidates for promotion. Zinc is present in almost all human tissues and in close to one hundred different enzymes in the body, and it plays an important role in growth processes. Calcium, in turn, is the body's most prevalent mineral and the major constituent of bone. It is also essential for maintaining cell membranes, proper blood clotting, and other important functions.

Purportedly, any ill that may befall the human organism might be related to a deficiency of one or both of these crucial minerals. At least, that's what food-fad promoters would like you to think. The facts are somewhat different.

Zinc is plentiful in the ordinary American diet, especially in meat and other animal proteins. Accordingly, anyone who eats a balanced variety of foods is unlikely to become deficient in zinc. A problem may arise among people who eat little or no animal protein, particularly if their diet is high in cereal grains. Whole grains contain zinc, but some of them—especially wheat—also contains phytates, agents that can bind metals such as zinc and make them unavailable for absorption by the body. Unleavened bread appears to be a particular problem in this regard. Certain diseases, such as cirrhosis of the liver, may also result in increased urinary loss of body zinc. But most healthy

Americans eating typical diets needn't worry about a shortage of zinc.

The versatile role of calcium in the body often prompts self-styled nutrition seers to warn about endless miseries that might result from a lack of this mineral. Bleeding problems, menstrual cramps, insomnia, muscle spasms, and indigestion supposedly await the laggard calcium ingester. Bone meal, dolomite, and other commercial calcium preparations are touted to ward off such consequences.

None of those ills results from a calcium deficiency. The bones serve as an enormous calcium reservoir for the body. Under hormonal influence, they continually lose and regain calcium to keep its level stable in the blood and other body fluids. If a diet is deficient in the calcium, the bones may suffer, but the role of calcium in intricate metabolic reactions and functions will be preserved. Moreover, taking a calcium supplement won't necessarily prevent a deficiency. Calcium balance in the body is significantly affected by the intake of protein and phosphorus as well as that of calcium. It's the overall diet that's important, not just separate components of it.

What about so-called organic foods? There's nothing inherently wrong with them. If they are marketed close to their source of origin and are fresh and tasty, some people may prefer them to a conventionally marketed product. But are they more nutritious or better for your health than ordinary fare?

Promoters of organic foods apparently would like you to think so. They stress the point that foods labeled "organic" are supposed to be produced without the aid of synthetic fertilizers or pesticides and without using preservatives or other chemicals in their preparation. The implication is that such foods are likely to be better for you and presumably worth the premium prices commonly charged for them. (Surveys comparing prices of organic and conventional foods consistently show much higher prices for organic foods—whether sold in health food stores or in the "organic" section of supermarkets.) The implication of health benefits, however, has little basis in fact.

One of the alleged advantages, for instance, is that organic foods are produced without pesticides. But that doesn't mean such foods are free of pesticide residues. According to the FDA, analyses of many organic foods show minute traces of pesticides, just as many conventional foods do. Some residues remain in the soil years after the last pesticide application, and fresh residues may be deposited by drifting sprays and dusts or by rainfall runoff from nearby farms. A study by the New York State Food Laboratory in 1972 found that products labeled "organic," which were purchased at health food stores by government agents, showed pesticide residues at least as often as regular foods tested at the same laboratory.

Nor are foods grown with natural fertilizers, such as manure, any more nutritious than conventionally grown crops. Organic fertilizers cannot be used directly by a plant. They must first be broken down by soil bacteria into inorganic compounds. The inorganic compounds actually taken up by the plant are identical to those supplied directly by synthetic fertilizers.

The vitamin content of plants is determined primarily by their heredity. Vitamins are manufactured by the plants themselves through genetically controlled processes. They are not taken up by the plant from the soil. In contrast, the mineral content of a plant is dependent on the mineral content of the soil. However, if soil is deficient in certain trace minerals, adding fertilizer from the same farm or locale would be an inefficient way to restore those minerals because the local fertilizer is likely to be deficient in them as well.

The promotional value of excluding preservatives or similar agents from organic foods is not automatically matched by any health value. An organic bread made without the common preservative calcium propionate might sound chemically pure. But an ounce of Swiss cheese on the bread will add enough calcium propionate to preserve two loaves of bread. It occurs naturally in Swiss cheese. Presumably, bread isn't made any safer by omitting a natural substance not known to be harmful. But it may get moldy faster.

The extra outlay of money for organic foods or dietary nostrums is usually the only loss suffered by buyers. But when nutrients are used in large doses as medicines, there's always the possibility of an adverse reaction. Two incidents publicized in recent years illustrate what can sometimes happen.

According to a case report in *The Journal of the American Medical Association,* the parents of a two-month-old boy gave the child a large dose (3 grams) of potassium chloride, a common salt substitute, as a remedy for "colic." The treatment, which had been recommended in the book *Let's Have Healthy Children* by the late nutritionist Adelle Davis, resulted in the infant's death. The parents are suing the publisher of the book and Davis's estate for damages in excess of $1 million.

A second incident reported in *JAMA* involved a California woman whose acting career ended when she developed an incapacitating illness. After more than twenty physicians failed to find the cause, the woman finally made the diagnosis herself. An investigation of the medical literature convinced her that she was suffering from lead poisoning. Subsequent testing revealed that she was right.

The source of the lead was a bone-meal supplement that the woman had been taking for six years. Analysis showed significant levels of lead in the health food product, which was made from horse bones. The bone meal contained 190 parts per million of lead, more than twenty times the average content that the FDA has found in similar products made from cattle bones.

Serious side effects from taking large doses of certain vitamins, minerals, or other health food preparations are not rare occurrences. What is rare about the experiences suffered by the infant and the actress is that they received press coverage. The involvement of a popular nutritionist's book and the human interest aspect of a patient's discovery of what her doctors had missed made both incidents especially newsworthy.

Comparable reports appear every so often in medical journals, but only a few receive wide exposure. Indeed, the report concerning the infant death from potassium chloride actually described two fatalities. The other was that of a thirty-two-year-old woman who died of an overdose of potassium chloride, which she reportedly took indiscriminately whenever she felt weak or tired. Her death was unrelated to the Adelle Davis book, however, and has received little further publicity.

As the potassium chloride deaths indicate, even a relatively common food substance can be dangerous when misused. Several essential vitamins and minerals —vitamins A and D, iron, selenium, and calcium—can all be toxic in large doses. Excessive amounts of vitamin D, for example, may retard growth in children and can also increase the blood calcium level, causing vomiting, constipation, kidney stones, and even death.

Calcium, which is required in relatively large quantities by the body, can also cause adverse effects in excessive doses. Too much of it may produce symptoms similar to vitamin D toxicity. Severe side effects have also occurred among people taking large amounts of vitamin A. And a variety of adverse effects have now been reported with megadoses of vitamin C, which was once thought to be relatively harmless in such amounts. At present, the most commonly noted side effect from large doses of vitamin C is diarrhea. But some individual case reports suggest that such doses may in certain instances lead to kidney problems, adverse effects on the fetus, development of vitamin B-12 deficiency, and interference with some antidepressant medications. Experiments with animals have also raised speculation about possible detrimental effects of large doses of vitamin C on growing bone.

Some health food staples can also be hazardous. Certified raw milk, for example, has been linked by California health officials to numerous cases of Salmonella dublin infection, a form of food poisoning that can be severe or even fatal, especially among elderly or sick people. As already noted, some bone meal derived from horses may contain high levels of lead. Kelp tablets may contain high levels of iodide and arsenic. Various herb teas contain chemical compounds that may cause adverse effects ranging from mild to severe. According to *The Medical Letter,* a nonprofit publication for medical professionals that evaluates drugs and other substances, herb teas containing buckthorn bark, senna leaves, dock roots, or aloe leaves may cause severe diarrhea. Burdock tea may cause blurred vision, inability to void, and bizarre behavoir and speech. Nutmeg tea may cause severe headache, cramps, and nausea. Tea made from chamomile flower heads may cause contact dermatitis, allergic shock, or other severe hypersensitivity reactions in people allergic to ragweed or similar pollens. "Herbal teas may have only a single ingredient or may be blends of as many as 20 different kinds of leaves, seeds, and flowers," *The Medical Letter* noted. "Few buyers are aware of the potential dangers of some of these products."

In short, the use of some foods or beverages as medicine may present the kinds of hazards ordinarily associated with a drug or medication. The fact that something is identified as a food or vitamin does not render it harmless in excessive amounts.

Recommendations

While food-fad nostrums won't prevent or cure disease, good nutrition is still essential to overall health. The basics of sound nutrition aren't as complicated as people are sometimes led to believe. If anything, the trouble with good nutrition is that it's fairly straightforward and unexciting—not the stuff that best-sellers are made of.

The common recommendation to eat a variety of foods has a sound reason behind it. If you eat a varied and well-balanced diet, you're likely to get all of the nutrients you need and not too much of any one substance that might be detrimental. Admittedly, the heavy promotion of many high-calorie, low-nutrient products by food manufacturers can get in the way of selecting a proper diet. So it can take some conscious effort to achieve good nutrition.

A useful guide is to include some choices daily from each of the four main food groups: the milk group (milk, cheese, yogurt, and other dairy foods); the meat group (meat, poultry, fish, eggs, and meat alternatives such as dried beans, lentils, and nuts); the bread group (bread, cereal, noodles, rice, and other grain products); and the vegetable group (vegetables and fruit).

A balanced diet—one that supplies enough calories, protein, vitamins, and minerals for the body's needs—can generally be achieved by favoring unprocessed foods and including two or more servings daily from each of the four main food groups. There's nothing sacred about the "basic four," though. It's simply convenient for the food customs of most Americans. A different combination can be worked out for those who choose a strict vegetarian diet, provided they include a source of vitamin B-12, which is rarely found in plant foods.

Finally, don't worry if you don't eat a balanced diet every day. CU's medical consultants believe it's long-term balance that's important, and even several days of erratic eating are unlikely to have any significant effect on your health.

Afterword

As this book has demonstrated, three federal agencies —the U.S. Food and Drug Administration, the Federal Trade Commission, and the U.S. Postal Service—play a part in the battle to curtail health quackery. But even all three agencies, acting in concert, cannot assure that the public will be adequately protected. Nor can people necessarily count on the medical profession to unmask questionable practitioners who operate under the cloak of official licensure.

Although machinery exists for depriving physicians who are incompetents or charlatans of their right to practice medicine, the procedures are so cumbersome that they are seldom invoked. The authority to hear charges and, theoretically, to revoke licenses is delegated to state and county medical societies. These bodies are often content merely to reprimand a physician brought up on charges. The physician, duly reprimanded, is then usually permitted to resume normal practice.

Afterword

Unless the role of government agencies in the prevention of health frauds is substantially strengthened and unless there are more stringent penalties for abuses of medical privilege, the most reliable bulwark against health quackery is a vigilant consumer. If you suspect that a treatment or cure suggested to you by an advertisement, a book, a friend, or a relative may be fraudulent, you may be able to obtain helpful answers to questions from a number of organizations. (Most of these organizations appreciate being notified of questionable activity in their areas of special interest.) Some of the places to try are:

☐American Cancer Society, The Unproven Methods of Cancer Management Committee, 777 Third Avenue, New York, New York 10017. (212) 371–2900.

☐American Dental Association, Council. on Dental Therapeutics, 211 East Chicago Avenue, Chicago, Illinois 60611. (312) 440–2527.

☐American Medical Association, Archive Library, 535 North Dearborn Street, Chicago, Illinois 60610. (312) 751–6000.

☐Arthritis Foundation, Lenox P.O. Box 1888, Atlanta, Georgia 30326. Attention: Medical Department. You can also telephone one of the seventy-two local chapters.

☐Consumer Product Safety Commission, Bethesda, Maryland 20016. In continental United States—except Maryland—(800) 638–8326. In Maryland (800) 492–8363. In Alaska, Hawaii, Puerto Rico, Virgin Islands (800) 638–8333.

☐Federal Trade Commission, Bureau of Consumer

Protection, Division of Food and Drug Advertising, Washington, D.C. 20580.

□U.S. Food and Drug Administration, Consumer Inquiry/Complaints, Rockville, Maryland 20857. (301) 443–3170. The FDA's district offices are listed under Health, Education, and Welfare Department in telephone directories for the cities in which they are located.

□U.S. Postal Service, Special Investigation Division of Postal Inspection Service, 475 L'Enfant Plaza, S.W., Washington, D.C. 20260. For information and complaints about mail-order products (202) 245–4000. You can also reach the Postal Inspection Service through your local postmaster.

□Your state or local health department or medical society.

Finally, we invite readers of *Health Quackery* who have comments about the book, experiences to share, or information to impart to write to us at Consumer Reports Books, 256 Washington Street, Mount Vernon, New York 10550.

Index

Index

Index

Index

Index

Index